Redefining Aging

Redefining Aging

A CAREGIVER'S GUIDE TO
LIVING YOUR BEST LIFE

Ann Kaiser Stearns, PhD

Foreword by J. Raymond DePaulo, Jr., MD

Johns Hopkins University Press • Baltimore

Note to the Reader: This book is not meant to substitute for medical care and treatment should not be based solely on its contents. Instead, treatment must be developed in a dialogue between the individual and his or her physician. Our book has been written to help with that dialogue.

© 2017 Johns Hopkins University Press
All rights reserved. Published 2017
Printed in the United States of America on acid-free paper
9 8 7 6 5 4 3 2 1

Johns Hopkins University Press
2715 North Charles Street
Baltimore, Maryland 21218-4363
www.press.jhu.edu

Library of Congress Cataloging-in-Publication Data

Names: Stearns, Ann Kaiser, author.
Title: Redefining aging : A caregiver's guide to living your best life
    / Ann Kaiser Stearns, PhD.
Description: Baltimore : Johns Hopkins University Press, [2017] | Includes bibliographical
    references and index.
Identifiers: LCCN 2017007362| ISBN 9781421423678 (hardcover : alk. paper) |
    ISBN 1421423677 (hardcover : alk. paper) | ISBN 9781421423685 (pbk. : alk.
    paper) | ISBN 1421423685 (pbk. : alk. paper) | ISBN 9781421423692
    (electronic) | ISBN 1421423693 (electronic)
Subjects: LCSH: Caregivers. | Older people—Care. | Care of the sick—
    Psychological aspects. | Consumer education.
Classification: LCC RC108 .S74 2017 | DDC 362.1084/6—dc23
    LC record available at https://lccn.loc.gov/2017007362

A catalog record for this book is available from the British Library.

Special discounts are available for bulk purchases of this book. For more information, please contact Special Sales at 410-516-6936 or specialsales@press.jhu.edu.

Johns Hopkins University Press uses environmentally friendly book materials, including recycled text paper that is composed of at least 30 percent post-consumer waste, whenever possible.

In memory of my mother,
Margaret O. Kaiser

And to honor my daughters,
Amanda Asha and Ashley Anjali

We realize that life
is so much a matter
of walking in gardens
and learning to recognize
that a garden is where we are.

—Ann Kaiser Stearns

Contents

Chapter 7. Comforting Insights and Myth-Busting Knowledge   113

Chapter 8. You're Not a Bad Person Because You're   128
Exhausted or Just Need a Life of Your Own

Chapter 9. Truly Helpful Caregiving Tips   150

Chapter 10. When Your Loved One Dies—   164
Relief, Grief, and Moving Forward

Foreword

Professor Ann Kaiser Stearns has written a wonderful and, at least to me, a surprising book. I was expecting a book about one thing, the terrible difficulties that confront caregivers (75 percent of whom are women) and a practical approach to managing them, and this book delivers on this count. But there are two distinct parts of the story that I hadn't expected, although I should have expected that a part of the book would be about grieving. First, the loss of a soul mate who is still alive but not able to connect in that soulful way anymore is a painful reality. Most of us who have been caregivers are unprepared for this loss, and I suspect that many deal with it (as I did) in fits and starts. Second, and surprising for me, is the book's significant reflection on how to use the experience of caregiving to consider your own future, including when you will need care later in life.

The book deals explicitly with the medical risks of being a sole caregiver without support: preventing one's own debilitation to the extent possible, even diminishing to some degree the risk of developing Alzheimer's disease oneself. This reflection on the aging caregiver may have been the wellspring for the title of the book. Dr. Stearns places a kind but clear emphasis on recognizing the many limits that all of us, but especially caregivers, face. Several chapters are here to remind you that providing your future caregivers with options and a recognition that they will need support for themselves is a very good idea, if and when they become your caregivers. From this important idea comes her epilogue to her two daughters and the book's subtitle: *A Caregiver's Guide to Living Your Best Life.*

I read books slowly and my engagement is always with the author, not just the book I am reading. This is a quintessential Ann Kaiser Stearns piece of writing: optimistic, warm, forward looking, and practical. As a college professor who also frequently gives presentations to other helping professionals and laypeople, Dr. Stearns has high expectations and standards but is full of generosity and a passion for her work. As an author, she brings these same qualities to this readable, compassionate approach to a journey most of us will take.

J. Raymond DePaulo, Jr., MD
University Distinguished Service Professor
Department of Psychiatry and Behavioral Sciences
Johns Hopkins University School of Medicine

Preface

You may be living with and caring for an older adult family member day in and day out, or you may be overseeing care for your loved one from across town or across the country. Whatever your experience as a caregiver, this book will help you find the best life within reach for *both* of you. Even if your elderly spouse, parent, or other family member is significantly impaired, there are good quality of life experiences still possible for him or her and for you.

As hard as it may seem now, it *is* possible to take good care of yourself and live a meaningful life while coping with the high stress, many challenges, and exasperating problems you're having to deal with—and this book will show you how. I think you will be uplifted and strengthened by the lessons learned and stories shared here by family caregivers who have faced their own tough situations. From my personal experience and extensive research, as well as that of many other professionals, I can promise you encouraging and comforting insights, empowering knowledge, and a host of problem-solving strategies. Along the way and in each appendix, you'll also learn about the available resources for support that you may need now or later on.

There are many psychological and emotional challenges of caregiving that most other books on elder care don't address, and that is why I've written this book. Chronic stress, grief, anger, guilt, and (most especially) anxiety about our own aging are feelings and concerns most caregivers have to deal with in order to lead rewarding lives and not become burned out. As hard as it is to believe this when you're battling fatigue and feeling stretched thin physically, emotionally, or financially, you can grow stronger and lead a richer life while being a caregiver to your loved one and be at peace after his or her passing.

You'll find here the stories of caregivers who have surely struggled and felt overwhelmed at times, but who have found ways to meet the challenges they faced, behaved bravely, and found a deep sense of purpose in caregiving. I think of them as inspiring role models. This book will also help you think constructively about how to take better care of yourself, reduce your own risk factors for Alzheimer's disease and other forms of dementia, and age as successfully as you can. You'll be helped to plan ahead for making life easier and more rewarding for the persons most likely to take care of *you* in your elder years. And to help you as you face your loved one's or your own aging, there are other inspiring stories of people showing us how to grow old well—still finding the best life within reach.

Acknowledgments

A special expression of appreciation is owed to Jacqueline Wehmueller, my editor at Johns Hopkins University Press: until Jackie reached out to me more than three years ago with the first idea for this book, I hadn't realized what a compelling need exists for this practical guidebook to encourage and support those who have an elderly loved one in need of caregiving. Three wise and wonderful friends, each with good judgment and noteworthy professional experience, gave invaluable advice and feedback on every chapter: to Judith V. Douglas, Marian Wattenbarger, and the Reverend Mary Gaut, I will always be thankful for the ways each made me a stronger writer, a better human being, and a more effective helping professional. Jonathan Norton, my former college student (now at Yale University), helped me track down and organize more than 500 research articles. Linda J. Walter helped greatly with copyediting. Joann Munden, my personal assistant and our family helper for 27 years, made my long work hours possible and rewarding: without her, I couldn't have raised my girls as a single parent or written this book and others. Similarly, Blake and Marian Wattenbarger—faithful and supportive godparents to my daughters, and my cherished friends since college—have helped to make my life richer and smoother as a parent, happier as a person, and more productive as an author and helping professional: they are the second set of siblings God gave me.

Other close friends upon whom I've long been able to rely for encouragement, good ideas, fun times, and warm support include Robbe and Keith Pohl, Charlie Metz, Melissa Hopp and Jody Bauer, Cherry and Lorenzo Marquez, Burt and Linda English, Kim Ward, Ron Potter, Lenny and Judy Mancini, Jan and Ron Allen, and the late Dorris Hoyle and her family. My neighbors Jane and Al Budacz also were constant sources of encouragement. Two other friends kept me physically strong: athletic trainer Anne Currie and physical therapist Cindy Chapman Hoerl. Fellow Baltimore Orioles baseball fans, including walking buddies Mary Jo Zimmer and Jeannie Clancy helped, too, and card-playing friends Jean and Jack Smith, Marsha Carroll, Betty Scott, Val Guperlet, and others mentioned above. Certified financial planner Chris Walker shared valuable financial advice, while Bonnie Travieso, Esq., contributed her legal knowledge. At the Community College of Baltimore County, where I teach full time, Dean Tim Davis and President Sandra Kurtinitis have been particularly supportive of this project. My academic vice president and the board of trustees joined them in approving a yearlong sabbatical.

Our border collie, Panda, kept her sweet furry self near my desk as I wrote and repeatedly rewrote the book. My dear daughters were supportive while Amanda completed her master's degree, Ashley planned her wedding, and new son-in-law, Chris, helped out with odd jobs involving a ladder and roof climbing.

I am grateful to have had amazing mentors and inspiring professors at Oklahoma City University, Duke University, the University of Edinburgh, the Union Institute and University, and in my clinical training in psychology at the Johns Hopkins University Medical Center and the Washington Pastoral Counseling Center. I'm thankful for Dr. J. Raymond DePaulo's publications, medical seminars, and encouragement of my work over the years. I am thankful, too, for countless other learning opportunities and for the love relationships I've been blessed to have. My life is also richly blessed for having had a loving mother and grandmother, and having a meaningful lifetime of work, loving daughters, and good friends.

And last—but certainly not least—I am grateful to the many caregivers who opened their hearts and shared their lives with me in order to help you, the reader, with your caregiving journey. I'm thankful for what I've learned from them, from my own parents and grandmother in their elder years, and from the remarkable researchers and authors whose knowledge shared here will empower you. All of the stories are true, but many of the names of people I interviewed for the book and the names of their family members have been changed to pseudonyms.

Redefining Aging

The Challenge

It is not only medicine that is needed in one's declining years but life—
a life with meaning, a life as rich and full as possible under the
circumstances.
    —Oliver Sacks, reviewing the book *Being Mortal*,
    by physician-author Atul Gawande

I have spent my career as a psychologist studying how people become resilient, able to stand strong, and live rewarding lives, despite hurtful, often devastating losses and other difficult life events. This time, I'm writing about the many ways it's still possible to be resilient—grow stronger, wiser, and even healthier—while dealing with the high stress of providing care for your impaired and elderly parent, spouse, or other family member. Alongside the many challenges and hardships, being a caregiver can add purpose to your life and increase your level of personal well-being and happiness.

The person in your care may be physically ill or disabled, cognitively impaired, or simply growing old and frail. It's true that more than 5 million Americans suffer from Alzheimer's disease, and hundreds of thousands more are afflicted with other types of dementia due to having severe strokes, head injuries, or other illnesses. But it's also true that there are many who are just wearing down with old age and the illnesses that often accompany it. In fact, 50 percent of Americans still don't have dementia at age 85.

You may find yourself with a seemingly endless emergence of problems to solve and countless emotions to work through, including fatigue, frustration, anxiety, depression, and feelings of guilt or resentment. Such feelings are often part of a grief and healing process that can begin before a person dies. You may also feel a deep sense of loss. It's hard to watch this person who lived an active and independent life become increasingly fragile and reliant on others for protection and care. Whether your loved one wants to stay in his or her own home, now lives with you, or resides in a care facility, you know that it's even harder for him or her to live with so much vulnerability.

Your brain may be bursting with concerns and questions: Are the memory lapses I'm seeing in my elderly parent or spouse due to problems often associated with aging, such as a treatable biochemical depression or other medical illness, the side effect of medicines, or vision or hearing loss? Are they caused by alcohol abuse? Or are they actually signs of dementia? How can I tell the difference between the cognitive impairments associated with normal aging and those due to early Alzheimer's disease? How do I respond to repetitive storytelling and the same questions asked again and again, frustration over episodes of forgetfulness, or resistance to the idea of giving up driving? Why does my loved one seem to be doing so well one day then, on the next day, show these odd episodes of being suspicious, angry, or disoriented? Am I witnessing some kind of personality changes that we all just have to accept? Is there anything I can do that will make things better?

At times the challenges are heartbreaking when you are caring for an elderly loved one with many medical issues, who may also struggle with increasing dependency, a diminishing quality of life, and a lessening sense of privacy. But for many caregivers there isn't time for heartbreak and tending to your own grief, especially if you are heavily burdened with the tasks of providing physical care or dealing with the behavioral problems of an elder with dementia. For example, you can feel drained of all energy when you have to overrule your mother's decisions because her memory and thinking are impaired or she is having a bad reaction to a medication. It may become a necessary way of dealing with exhaustion (and so many problems to solve) to close down your feelings, at least for a period of time. Focusing on making decisions and solving problems can be the only way it's possible to cope.

Whether your loved one scarcely has the means to make ends meet or you fear that resources might not last to the end of their life, money is a worry to most people. Along with everything else, there are safety concerns. It's important to you that your frail elder be treated with kindness and respect. You worry about your loved one's susceptibility to negligence and physical, mental, financial, or sexual abuse from paid caregivers or even other family members. The statistics are shocking as to how many caregivers (once thought trustworthy) *admit* to manipulating, mistreating, or abusing a vulnerable elderly person.[1] And many of us blame ourselves, thinking that our failure to protect our loved one was a kind of abuse, and feeling that we could have, or should have, done more than we did.

Take heart. Most problems have solutions: there are ways to provide for your loved one's protection, gain relief by finding answers to many of your troublesome concerns, and learn more about available resources for guidance and support. Caring, competent, affordable help can be found despite limited financial resources, and I'll share some ways to find it in later chapters.

Holocaust survivor and physician Viktor Frankl wrote, "Emotion which is suffering ceases to be suffering once a clear and precise picture is formed of it."[2] Despite times of despairing and feeling overwhelmed, there are new ways of thinking and actions to take that will make your life feel much better and your loved one's life better, too.

A BLESSING OR A BURDEN?

In the following chapters in this book, I'll be looking deeply into the many stories I've gathered from family members coping with the burdens and experiencing the blessings of caregiving. In their stories are insights and healing concepts that can make you stronger.

Many, many women and men provide loving care to their life partner or parent in old age, and I am writing for everyone who has a caregiving role. We enjoy the rewards of the loving relationships we've nurtured over the years but frequently feel pulled in many directions. Although in all North American ethnic groups, 75 to 80 percent of caregivers are women, men the world over also provide loving, graceful, dedicated care.

Even though our will to provide care for our elderly loved one may be very strong and deeply rewarding because of the closeness we share, most likely there will be times when we find caregiving exhausting, experience resentment, or feel burned out in other ways. Especially if our loved one has dementia and problems arise, such as a sudden onset of agitation, wandering, or accusing family members of stealing, strategies are needed to handle these situations. Specific problems like these require a plan of action to modify the environment that triggers the troublesome behavior—skills helpful to both the caregiver and the care recipient, ways of coping that can be learned from reading this book as well as other books and resources I will recommend. Researchers from the Johns Hopkins University School of Medicine and Utah State University found that elders with dementia have a "notably slower decline in both cognition and function" when caregivers regularly use "problem-focused coping [which] consists of seeking solutions coupled with formulating and implementing a plan of action to address the source of a problem."[3]

Even in the midst of a caregiving crisis, there are ways to cope—if you understand that being a caregiver can be a blessing or a burden or both at the same time. The heavy load of caregiving can be made lighter. A problem-solving approach will empower you while just hoping for things to get better will gradually weigh you down. Looking after an elderly family member typically lasts about a decade, and chronic stress can take its toll on your mental and physical health.[4] If your loved one has advanced dementia, you may find that gradually you are emotionally withdrawing from her or him, while still remaining kind and seeing to your elderly impaired person's high-quality care. Using detachment (consciously or unconsciously) as a coping mechanism may be necessary to your psychological survival when you've had a close relationship with this spouse, parent, grandparent, or sibling whose deterioration you find unbearably painful.[5] You aren't a bad person if detachment helps you to protect yourself and carry on with your other relationships and responsibilities. Perhaps you grieved earlier or will mourn after your loved one dies.

Soldiering on without support from family or community resources is a stress that can wear you down. Some of the caregivers I spoke with when I was writing this book told me that they initially didn't look for help not just because they thought they should cope on their own but also because they simply didn't know where to look. Later, when I tell you their stories, you'll learn some of the places they, sometimes to their surprise, found support.

An enormous body of research underlies the adage that "it is more blessed to give than to receive." Helping others (as in doing volunteer work or caring for a loved one who has suffered a stroke) can improve your physical strength and overall sense of well-being, decrease feelings of anxiety and depression, increase life satisfaction, and lengthen longevity.[6] Studies also show, however, that bearing the load of chronic stress without the relief of getting time for yourself (as in the so-called 36-hour-day of providing care for a loved one with dementia) can *decrease* life satisfaction and *increase* your risk of health problems, anxiety and depression, burnout, and even a shortened life.[7]

Of course, providing care for your frail spouse, parent, or other elderly family member does not have to threaten your health. Even what David Roth, at the Johns Hopkins University School of Medicine, calls "high-strain caregiving" can be rewarding if you learn ways to handle highly stressful situations effectively or avoid them altogether. Dr. Roth goes further and suggests that the benefit of successful caregiving may not be limited to those receiving the care—it may even reduce the risk of death for caregivers.[8] Experiences of caregiving that involve love, empathy, and "a sense of meaning or mattering" have been shown in studies to promote health, reduce stress, and decrease mortality.[9]

Whether caregiving is experienced as burdensome or meaningful also is related to how many hours per week one devotes to caregiving and whether significant time is invested in other activities, too. In what is described as an "eye-catching finding," researchers at the Nordic College of Caring Science report that "persons who combine caregiving with a paid job or voluntary work are *happier* than persons who are only engaged in caregiving or not engaged in any activities."[10]

One thing I know is true: Many of the people I have interviewed for this book insist that looking after their loved one, despite its heartbreaks, gave their own life greater meaning. For some, it was a way to give back the love they had been given. For others, caring for the very person who failed to be the good partner or parent they wished for allowed them to grow, rise above old resentments, and "move beyond what was broken."

CAREGIVING: A CHALLENGE AT ANY AGE

Because Americans are living so much longer, you may be a "young old" person (65+) with the challenging responsibilities of taking care of your "old old" (80–85+) family member.[11] At the other end of the caregiver continuum, if you are in your 20s or 30s or 40s, your battle to overcome the hardships and chronic stress of caregiving is possibly even greater than if you were yourself a senior citizen. If you allow it to do so, attending to the needs of your elderly family member without also carving out time for pursuing your own goals can rob you of your dreams. What can you do to keep yourself from being overwhelmed by the stress of caregiving? For starters, you can recognize that you are not alone; there are others who have faced and found ways to overcome the same challenges. So can you.

If you were born between 1946 and 1964, the chances are very high that you have been, are now, or soon will be responsible for the care and protection of an aging parent or other family member. A baby boomer, you are one of 80 million US adults in your 50s, 60s, or heading into your 70s while facing one of life's most taxing unpaid occupations. As a member of the "sandwich generation," you're probably trying to help out your adult children, grandchildren, or nieces and nephews while you provide care for your mentally or physically impaired spouse or parent.

Regardless of your age, if you are like most adult children or spouses, you are helping your impaired elderly loved one willingly but still find the caregiving stressful. The same is likely to be true if the family member in your care is a sibling, aunt, uncle, or grandparent.

While trying to do right by your loved one, you are presented with a huge challenge. You probably find yourself with "role overload"—too many responsibilities and decisions to make, including handling conflicting loyalties and competing emotions. You may have an adult child or other close family member in another part of the country who needs your help but feel at wits' end as to who would care for your elderly spouse or parent in your place here at home.

Even without conflicts of this kind, some of the signs of caregiver stress that you may be experiencing include fatigue, moodiness or a low-grade depression, forgetfulness, impatience, accident proneness, difficulty concentrating, feelings of guilt or resentment, and aches and pains of various kinds. Caregiver stress also can be expressed in the form of sleep disturbances, loss of appetite or overeating, too much television watching, or a general increase in health problems of your own. Understanding that these are *symptoms*—and that symptoms have remedies—is a first step toward dealing with the stress that causes them. Another step in the right direction is not to fall prey to excessive worry about the future—worry that may in fact be a *cause* of our stress, not just a symptom of it.

"If you are a zebra running for your life," writes Robert Sapolsky in *Why Zebras Don't Get Ulcers*, "your body's physiological response mechanisms are superbly adapted for dealing with such short-term physical emergencies."[12] But we aren't zebras running from a real and present danger. We're human beings, worrying about what hasn't happened yet or what might never happen but might . . . maybe not right now, maybe not this week, maybe not this month, but sometime in the future. Thankfully, there are stress-reducing activities we can learn (in chapter 6) to put an end to many of these self-induced, torturous worries about things that will never come to pass. We can take steps to greatly reduce the chronic excessive worrying that contributes to high blood pressure and heart disease.

The stress of caring for a loved one often overpowers even the caregiver's most valiant efforts to focus on the present. Over time the elderly person's impairments get worse and the ordeal of grief, caregiving, and problem solving worsens significantly. Dealing with memory problems and helping with medicines, transportation, shopping, and food preparation are challenges aplenty. Even more difficult is the huge task of finding kind ways to respond to our loved one's tears or confusion, paranoia or night terrors, wandering or screaming, inappropriate sexual behavior, hitting or verbal anger outbursts. The more troubling your loved one's behavior problems become, the more likely you are to struggle with a more severe form of depression, an illness that runs in families, especially if you or a close family member has suffered from an episode of major depression in the past.

In America, nearly one in four employed women and one in three unemployed women provide basic care for an aging parent. Two-thirds of all disabled elders are being cared for (10 to 20 hours a week) by a female family member, usually a daughter or daughter-in-law in her late 40s or early 50s who also has a full-time job. Ten percent of caregivers are working men, usually sons or sons-in-law, who provide care about 7 hours a week.[13] Many other family caregivers, especially spouses, average 20–40+ hours weekly.

Because so many unexpected difficulties arise, your job security may be suffering. You may be having problems with lateness and absenteeism or hurting financially because you've had to take a less demanding job, turn down a promotion, look for new employment after being let go, or give up working entirely.[14]

Unfortunately, your stress is apt to skyrocket if you quit your job to find enough time for elder care or if you are among the 23 percent of caregivers who once again share a home with your parent or parents.[15] While you now have more time for caregiving, there is apt to be more financial strain and alarmingly less time for your own adult relationships, recreational and educational interests, and the other activities (including exercise) that can effectively reduce stress. Work provides us with a reprieve from caregiving, gives us a variety of social contacts, and often enhances self-esteem. It's hard to replace these benefits when our world grows smaller.

As your level of involvement and the number of hours you invest in caregiving increase, what suffers is the time you spend with other family members and friends or pursuing hobbies, going on walks, or taking a vacation. All this adds up to more physical, emotional, financial, and role stress.[16]

There is hope, however. We know from research that helping your loved one in active ways can "make you physically stronger, improve your overall health, lift your spirits, and has even been shown to reduce mortality among caregivers."[17] Being actively helpful involves assisting with cooking meals, managing finances, helping your family member with getting in and out of bed or a chair, using the bathroom, and eating. Time spent providing this kind of help is less stressful and more uplifting than the "on-duty" time, when you are required (or feel you are) to stay nearby to make sure nothing goes wrong. Being constantly available and vigilant is taxing and burdensome because you are continuously required to be alert, never truly at rest, and you're unable to engage in the normal activities and routines of your own daily life.[18]

One of the hardest things to deal with is having your sleep interrupted time and again. Your elderly spouse or parent may wake up in the middle of the night and call out to you or get up and get dressed only to wander around the house or frighten you by suddenly standing over your bed! It is hard enough to cope with the high stress of caregiving on a good night's sleep, let alone when you're repeatedly sleep deprived. Leaving another family member in charge overnight or hiring someone familiar to your impaired loved one for overnight stays will allow you to get entirely away from on-duty time. Logging quality sleep on a regular basis is necessary to maintain not only your health but also your ability to handle the already plentiful challenges of caregiving.

Looking after your own needs is paramount. A red flag that says it is time to talk to your physician is any cluster of symptoms that may include fatigue, anxiety, difficulty concentrating, irritability or lashing out, a burdensome guilt, feelings of self-worthlessness or hopelessness, thoughts of death or suicide, a loss of pleasure in activities once satisfying, or an overwhelming feeling of sadness. Excessive alcohol use is another sign that professional help is needed. When a severely depressed or agitated mood persists and impairs your relationships or ability to sleep and function day to day, you probably have what we psychologists call "clinical" or major depression—a biochemical illness that usually needs to be treated with an antidepressant medication and supportive counseling. To lighten your load, you should ask about and utilize available elder care support services. Many of these resources are free from organizations like AARP (see appendix B), the National Alliance for Caregiving, and groups in your local community.

WHETHER SPOUSE OR PARENT—
FEELINGS OF LOSS OR RESENTMENT

Caregivers with a good-quality relationship before the illness onset feel less burdened than those whose relationship was not close.[19] But whether or not your prior relationship was fulfilling, experience shows that cutting back on your own personal activities to make time for your caregiving responsibilities leads to stress and distress.

If you are no longer able to participate in activities that you once shared with your loved one, you'll probably feel a sense of loss, both of the activity itself and of your former partner in it.[20] You may give up recreation outside the home that you used to enjoy, such as spending time with friends, and focus on caring for your spouse. If yours was a mutually loving relationship before you took on the role of caretaker, this sense of loss will inevitably be compounded by your concern for your partner's deteriorating health. If you've been blessed to have a good and loving life together, feelings of sadness and depression are unavoidable. Don't forget to care for yourself. There is comfort and strength to be found by engaging with family members and friends in the activities you miss most.

On the other hand, if your marriage relationship was *not* mutually giving or fulfilling, understandably your activity restriction is likely to leave you feeling resentful as well as depressed. What will help you to reduce your caregiver stress is to seek "assistance provided by others (e.g., friends, family members, service agencies) with caregiving tasks," so that you'll be less restricted and can resume the activities beneficial to you in the past. Taking better care of yourself, you may also be a kinder caregiver able to feel less resentful for your fate of taking care of a seriously ill spouse who was not especially responsive to your own needs in the past.[21]

These same principles and lessons apply to taking care of an impaired elderly parent or other relative with whom you were very close. You may find great meaning in being a loving caregiver. It will be sad, of course, and still have its challenges, but you will probably feel less burdened and have fewer stress symptoms. But if you are caring for someone with whom you have had a troubled, poor-quality relationship, you may experience greater stress and resent the burden that you are carrying.[22]

Getting emotional support from other family members, friends, neighbors, counselors, a clergy person, or from community agencies can benefit everyone, but especially the many caregivers who feel resentful. Support is needed whether or not you were close to your family member before he or she became old and impaired.

THE PERILS OF "JOHN HENRYISM"

In American folklore, John Henry was a railroad builder, a "steel driving man," determined, goal oriented, and strong. In an "epic battle of man against machine," he hammered a steel drill into rock at such a fast pace that he won a race against a steam-powered hammer. He prevailed over great odds, only to collapse and die from his efforts once he had completed his task. To many of us, he is a model of persevering through hard times and never giving up—even when circumstances are unbearable. Many people admire the enduring, steadfast family caretakers who go so far as to jeopardize their own health to look after their loved ones. We praise their "high effort coping in the face of adversity"— which just happens to be the definition of John Henryism.[23]

And you may expect the same of yourself. Caring for your aging spouse or parent, you may decide that you can cope if you are determined and work hard, that you can endure and move beyond the heartbreak and hardships you face. You may even think that admitting that the everyday stressors of caregiving are "just too much" would be a sign of weakness or mean that you are "giving in" or somehow failing as a person.

But long-term stress without relief takes its toll. You may not be like John Henry, who fell dead on the spot because of his exertions, yet your health may suffer over time. Despite some recent research to the contrary,[24] it seems to me to make sense that chronic stressors requiring a heavy burden of coping effort can exact a higher price for many people who are high on John Henryism (hard work and determination) but low on access to the resources they need to buffer their stress. And I am not alone in believing that trying to be John Henry can be hazardous to your health. According to an article in *Duke Medicine News and Communications*, "People with high levels of JH [John Henryism] and inadequate resources have a much higher prevalence of health disorders . . . because they drive themselves toward reaching specific goals at the expense of their health, often without realizing they are doing so."[25]

As a caregiver, you—perhaps more than anyone—*deserve* to have a self-care plan. Please take the time you need to come up with a list of specific ways to get respite time away from being "on call." Right now, get out a note pad. Write down the names of friends, family members, a coworker, or neighbor who would be willing to lend a hand—if you ask for an hour or a few here and there, on a certain day, days, or evening of the week. Jot down the activities you enjoy but haven't had time for, fun things that lift your spirits. Decide that your happiness and health matter. But *don't* use this time for shopping or house cleaning or doing laundry. Make your time away meaningful, relaxing, restorative, or fun: visit a friend, attend church or synagogue or your grandchild's school event, get out for exercise, see a movie, spend time in the sun reading a good book, gardening, knitting, or playing a sport. You can still be a good caregiver—in fact you'll become a *better*, more relaxed and effective caregiver by making time for yourself—and you'll feel happier, more able to experience feelings of satisfaction in your caregiving work. Whether you have trouble dealing with your impaired elder's problem behaviors or your own guilt, negative feelings, fatigue, and lack of even temporary relief from your tasks (or all of these), the challenges of caregiving often feel daunting. Even if you seem to be coping admirably, you may be growing increasingly worn down by your efforts, as your body weathers the assaults and trials associated with caring for your elderly loved one day after day. Taking care of yourself isn't a luxury, it's a necessity.

Fulfilling your role as a caregiver is more rewarding and may be less stressful if you are part of a family that respects and values the care of aging parents and other family members. Some cultures and subcultures are more supportive of family ties, traditions, and such loyalty. I hope you feel a sense of personal satisfaction and self-respect for the sacrifices you are making, the challenges you're taking on, and the kindness in your heart.

Many caregivers say that what helps them cope with the high stress of caregiving is "accepting change, getting help from professionals, releasing emotions and problem solving."[26] Many others describe the great benefit they receive from prayer and the support of their religious communities: religion gives strength by "[providing] a personal coping strategy and a social support network," both of which are exceedingly valuable in reducing stress. Also of importance to successful coping is "getting control" of difficult caregiving situations.[27]

Over my career, I have interviewed, taught, or counseled countless resilient people whose stories inspire me. Most of them have said they were strengthened by being determined to learn from their personal sorrows and challenges something of value to others. These "triumphant survivors," as I call them, often told me they were sustained by one or another form of spirituality: either trusting in a higher power or believing in moral values beyond themselves (such as service to others or the Golden Rule of treating others as we want to be treated). Making a decision to grow stronger, wiser, and more thankful for life itself—becoming a "better person" through adversity—is a meaningful strategy for coping with stress.

However strong and resilient you consider yourself to be, most of us in the medical and other helping professions agree: Working as a team with other family members who trade off the caregiving responsibilities, so that you don't have to bear the burden alone, will help you cope more effectively and feel psychologically stronger. To reduce the "higher levels of cortisol, indicating greater physiological stress," what is also needed is "tangible assistance, such as services, financial assistance, and other specific aid or goods, allowing [you] more time and energy."[28] With support, caregiving can give you a gratifying sense of satisfaction and self-respect.[29]

HAVING THE STRENGTH AND WISDOM
TO SEEK AND ACCEPT SUPPORT

Seventeen percent of Americans over age 75 need help with what are called instrumental activities of daily living, such as paying bills, doing housekeeping chores, shopping, and preparing meals. But what if helping with those is not enough? Where can you find help for your loved one's basic daily activities with which about 9 percent of elders have difficulty: getting up from a bed or chair, bathing, dressing, and eating?[30] What kinds of "respite interventions" are available so that you can reduce the time you spend on call, having to be on hand to keep your loved one safe or to handle problems that might arise? This "always on duty" situation is known to be especially burdensome. Thankfully, there are resources available that can give you back the time you need for your own recreational and spiritual activities and the relationships with others that sustain you and bring you joy.

Among other things, this book will suggest ways to tap online and community resources to help you choose a home health care provider, day care or memory care center, assisted living facility or nursing home. You will be guided to agencies that help people learn skills for dealing with difficult caregiving situations, help caregivers manage with limited financial resources, and give advice on how to monitor your loved one's care when it is provided by other family members or paid caregivers.

There are many coping strategies that you can employ to prevent caregiver burnout. To be healthy and stay well, acquiring some new skills and ways of thinking can help you understand, empathize with, respect, and interact positively with your elderly spouse or parent. A good starting place is to identify and put into your daily life, one at a time, the tried and proven stress-buffering activities that have worked well for you in the past.

For roughly one-half of caregivers who are taking care of a physically or cognitively disabled loved one, the experience turns out to be a challenging but deeply rewarding one. According to research on the subject, caregivers who find and use outside sources of support and seek solutions to problems are more able to find caregiving meaningful. Others who try to manage caretaking all on their own, without knowing about or having yet utilized resources for support, often describe the caretaking experience with exasperated expressions such as "feeling overwhelmed, spent, drowning." In the words of one caregiver of the sort none of us wants to be, "I'm like a rock already at the lake bottom!"

Being a caregiver can enrich your life by making your life deeply matter. You can grow stronger and wiser by allowing your eyes to see how the human spirit survives and thrives, even in a frail person who has had a debilitating stroke or is in the throes of Alzheimer's disease. This journey of giving your elderly spouse, parent, or other loved one the gift of respect and compassionate care will grow your self-respect. You can reap the benefits of becoming a better listener and kinder person. In the words of Professor William Haley, of the School of Aging at the University of South Florida, "People who find positive aspects of caregiving are not wearing rose colored glasses. It's a beneficial form of coping with stress."[31]

This book will offer a variety of helpful perspectives and innovative communication skills that can make your caregiving experience more personally fulfilling. Drawing from a wealth of academic research on these topics, my nearly four decades as a psychologist, and from other authors' books on caregiving, I will share with you the best of what I have learned—and I have had much to learn.

I especially look forward to sharing with you the insights I have mined from interviewing scores of family caregivers in their homes, talking with other professionals in my office or theirs, and visiting staff and residents in assisted living and nursing homes. In each of these settings, I have experienced a rich emotional exchange with family and professional caregivers and a meaningful connection on issues of the heart. I'll share, too, the role models on health and frailty given me by my own elderly grandmother and mother, whose strengths of character and wisdom prevailed despite the fact that each of them suffered from Alzheimer's disease prior to their deaths.

ANXIETY ABOUT OUR OWN AGING

All along the way, you will also be challenged to make some decisions that can make *your own old age* healthier and happier, one day enabling others to have a more positive experience taking care of *you*.

Caregiving triggers anxiety as we ponder our own aging, which greatly adds to our stress. Trying unsuccessfully not to look ahead, we fear losing our own independence and dignity. With horror, we imagine ourselves vulnerable and at the mercy of strangers, whether volunteers or paid caregivers. What will be my fate? Will I not recognize my own family members some day? We mutter within ourselves all sorts of such negative thoughts, in protest at life's unpredictability and potential cruelty. What if I am no longer seen as a person, no longer treated with respect? To our friends, life partner, or an adult child, we mumble or emphatically declare, "When I'm old, I'd rather *die* than be put in a nursing home!" And then, with a sigh of relief, we remember that at age 85 it is still the case that only about half of elders are suffering with dementia.

In calmer, more productive and grown-up conversations with ourselves, we ask, What kind of an old person will I be? Who will care for me? What decisions do I need to make and actions take to reduce my loved ones' caregiver stress when I need elder care? What can I do now to give my adult children fewer life complications later on as they provide for my care and hire others to help? In what ways can I grow into a nicer human being, to render it more likely that I'll be an old person able to receive care with grace and gratitude? Clearly, we realize, there are conversations we need to have with our partner, grown children, or other relatives about quality of life issues taking precedence over longevity, to inform their decisions about our end of life care.

All of us can avoid becoming "too soon old and too late smart," as Dr. Gordon Livingston puts it, quoting a Pennsylvania Dutch proverb in his thought-provoking book by that title. You can learn, as I have, from the resilient caregivers described in this book. You will see how is it possible to think in new ways about aging, to emulate the "old people" whose examples you hope to follow in health, illness, disability, and death. And finally, you can have the needed conversations about quality of life and other issues with those who may take care of *you* in the future.

We can each answer the challenge to manage our own aging in positive ways. There are lifestyle changes we can make that include behaviors and attitudes known to reduce or delay our risk of heart disease, strokes, and Alzheimer's disease. There are financial decisions and legal documents we can put in place, and ways each of us can grow to become the kind of person others will want to treat with respect and kindness when it's our turn to be elders so vulnerable and reliant on others.

There aren't any guarantees, of course. Things can and do happen to all of us beyond our control. Still, we've all known people in their elder years who have lived gracefully and gratefully, even with severe disabilities. We have an abundance of role models. Our challenge is to follow their lead.

On Both Sides, Vulnerability and Loss

We don't understand that we're going to parent our parents. I was shocked. I was honestly so blindsided by the entire experience of watching my parents' bodies fail that this movie is what came out of that.
—David Dobkins, director of *The Judge*

In her October 10, 2014, movie review written for *USA Today*, Andrea Mandell describes a scene in *The Judge* that made the award-winning actor Robert Duvall hesitate at first to accept the role he was offered: "It was a scene [where a frail old man needs his son's help to bathe] that nakedly portrays what it means to age (and be at the mercy of your grown child's care) that had Duvall turning away."

Whether it happens all at once because of a debilitating accident, illness, or stroke or gradually from a disease such as Parkinson's or Alzheimer's, we face a jolting realization. At some point, it dawns on us that *we* are now becoming our parent's parent, spouse's parent, grandparent or sibling's parent. It also dawns on us that—if we ourselves are lucky enough to grow old—someday we may be just as vulnerable and reliant on others to provide for *our* care.

There is an empathy and sadness that most of us feel for the person who was physically strong and self-sufficient and is now increasingly vulnerable, was independent and now needs help with the simple activities of daily life, was wise or skillful or not so much either but was always in control and now is unable to think through and solve many problems as mundane as paying bills or keeping track of which pills to take and when. We grieve for all that our loved one has lost, and he or she grieves, too, until severe dementia takes away the ability to sustain feelings of sorrow or regret.

Mourning is not just the process of grief and healing that takes place after a loved one dies. The word "bereavement" comes from the word "reave," which means to be dispossessed, robbed of something precious, something rightfully one's own.[1] Nothing belongs to us more than the human person we are and have always been! It is the greatest loss we can imagine for our loved one to bear and the greatest loss we fear having one day to bear ourselves.

Educator and author Laura E. Berk speaks of grief as "an unjust and injurious stealing of something valuable."[2] Although we don't like to think about it because we (wrongly) think there is no answer to being anxious about our own future vulnerability as elders, what is "stolen" is our sense of security. When we have to parent another adult, a family member who is now impaired but was once robust, we realize that the days of *our* being able to receive care from this person are over.

CARING FOR A SPOUSE

This loss is especially painful for those looking after a beloved partner. "For 15 years I cared for my Parkinson's spouse," wrote Diane Fasching, to the editor of the *AARP Bulletin*. "My husband and I went from equal partners to a dependent relationship." She wanted to emphasize "the need for the caregiver to obtain services, to fend off bitterness and to care for oneself."[3]

Another woman caring for her husband with Alzheimer's disease, in an interview with Anna Gorman of *Kaiser Health News*, said, "Part of what originally attracted me to Sid is that he was so intelligent, so quick minded. At times I have lost the person I married. He's just not the same."[4]

And it was true for the dad of a friend of mine, who was a devoted husband through the seven or eight years that his wife's Alzheimer's disease had its onset and gradually worsened. Mr. Salazar mostly loved her with kindness when she behaved in the ways people with dementia often behave. A notable exception was Mrs. Salazar's attachment to the same two outfits—the clothes she wanted to wear always and everywhere—because it was hard for him to get her into something else. Although it is extremely common for a person with dementia to cling to the security of a piece of clothing or other object, he got frustrated with his wife and she knew it.

Mr. Salazar also showed irritation when his wife of nearly 69 years was routinely slow getting dressed for church or for the metro-mobility bus that took her to a day care program. And it annoyed him that she never figured out how to operate the laundry machines that were available to them, just down the hall from their assisted living apartment. Even with the severe dementia that made it hard for Mrs. Salazar to understand many things in her daily world, her face showed that his impatience pained her. For her, the agitation and confusion of dementia often worsened at that moment of his expressed frustration.

"I just keep telling her and she doesn't get it!" Mr. Salazar would complain to his daughter. He thought if he said something often enough his wife would get it.

"You can't fight with someone with Alzheimer's so don't have a fight," my friend would say to her dad. Easier said than done, of course, because 24/7 caregiving is so stressful.

If you are in a similar caregiving situation, you may have questions on your mind such as these: With whom can I share the sadness I feel? In whom can I confide for comfort and strength? What promises did I make to my spouse or did we make to each other—"through sickness or in health . . . 'til death do us part"—and does that mean I have to be the primary caregiver? What if I'm getting old, too, feeling overwhelmed, and failing in strength? Where can I get needed support from resources in the community or other family members, and what activities can I engage in to buffer my stress?

Depending on your own health, the degree of your spouse's disability, and whether others are available to help when needed, you may find caregiving a challenge, even if it's not so sad or extremely stressful.

LOVING THE CHANGED SPOUSE

Reverend Mark is an 80-year-old man who does not have Alzheimer's disease but is suffering cognitive impairments from head injuries he received playing football years ago and more recently from falls on unexpectedly icy walkways. He often struggles to find the right words to complete a sentence. The former editor of a national publication and a retired clergyman with four master's degrees, Mark has given up teaching but is intelligent and engaging with loved ones who are patient and comfortable with filling in missing words. He and his wife, Laura, can enjoy a television show, sitting close and holding hands, if there is not too much dialogue and the story line isn't overly complex. Almost nightly he finds pleasure in watching televised reruns of shows from the 1960s and 1970s, especially *Hogan's Heroes* and *M*A*S*H*.

There are ways in which Mark's personality has changed that make Laura's caregiving difficult. His words can sound harsh and inflict hurt feelings if she doesn't quickly remind herself why Mark sometimes acts like an angry bear. After a lifetime of not being an aggressive or angry person, even these occasional times now when Mark is "gruff" keep surprising her, she says. "It all goes back to 1962," Laura explains. "As a young minister, assigned to a new church, Mark was playing football with boys from his youth group when he fell on blacktop and was knocked unconscious. He was hospitalized and his concussion symptoms lasted several days. As he was recovering and his brain was healing, Mark's doctor would not release him from the hospital because Mark was acting mean."

As the physician explained, "A minister can't act that way," especially not with a new congregation of people who haven't gotten to know him yet. "He has to get back to his regular self before I can let him go home," the doctor said.

Head injuries as well as Alzheimer's disease and other medical conditions often significantly alter the brain's ability to regulate emotions, leading to poor judgment, angry outbursts or inappropriate speech or behavior. Even in "normal" aging, when there is no dementia, our prefrontal cortex may function less well, meaning the part of our brain that is our CEO often isn't as sharp when we're making judgments, evaluating consequences, or keeping our emotional reactions in check.

Mark's long ago and more recent head injuries (his several concussions) began to have a cumulative effect in his late 70s. While his decision-making abilities are in good shape and he is physically stronger than most men 20 years younger, what is noteworthy are some speech and memory problems that trouble him greatly and some personality changes that Laura is sad to see. "There isn't much pretense about him anymore," Laura explains. "He doesn't try to be nice and is uncharacteristically blunt."

The CEO part of the human brain that acts as a filter to regulate emotions—enabling most of us to speak kindly at the appropriate time and carry a pleasant demeanor (regardless of how grumpy we might actually be feeling)—is one part of Mark's brain that is impaired now. For some odd reason, "if he's talking to someone on the phone, he can be very nice," Laura says, "but in person, his demeanor [again uncharacteristically] is often not pleasant." She has learned that what works best is to ignore his cranky comments. After all, there are many good things they continue to share, including a satisfying sex life, interesting visits with their children and grandchildren, religious services, their adult Sunday school class, and reruns of old TV sitcoms that bring smiles. Also cherished are the loving times when Mark tells Laura that *she* is the "main reason" that *he* has a life worth living.

When his head hit the pavement 50 years ago, Mark's young brain recuperated well because of what is described by neurologists today as "brain plasticity." Now the old injury plus subsequent concussions have caused his cognitive functioning and impulse-control problems to continue to worsen. "He is grumpy more often now," Laura says. She has to constantly remind herself not to take it personally when his comments are unkind. "It's his wounded brain talking," she has to tell herself. That's not the same husband she has known since they were college sweethearts.

For a time, while he was taking an antidepressant medication, Mark's somber mood lifted, and he seemed able to experience more pleasure in his daily life. Unfortunately, the antidepressant he was taking had sexual side effects so Mark quit taking it. With the exception of most geriatricians, many physicians seem to assume that elderly people aren't still having an active sex life. Maybe his doctor didn't ask about side effects or explain that other antidepressants could help his mood but not rob Mark and his wife of the intimacy and sexual fulfillment they've shared throughout their marriage. Depression is very common in elderly people, with or without dementia. But you can't fault an 80-year-old man for not wanting to jeopardize the pleasure he *is* able to enjoy and share with his wife, having lost the mental sharpness that gave him decades of pleasure as a scholar, theologian, author, and teacher.

Because his loving wife sees herself as simply returning to her husband the care, companionship, and protection that she received from him in their more than 50-year marriage, Laura is sad for him but not for herself. Mark has changed and she is willing to change, too. His memory keeps getting worse, and he often goes long periods without speaking. She loves him, accepts him as he is, and is thankful for all that Mark is still able to do: he exercises on a treadmill and lifts weights six days a week, still drives, still does all the yard work on their two-acre property and shovels snow, takes care of his own personal hygiene including choosing his clothes and dressing, and (like always) fixes his own breakfast and lunch. A key to their happiness is that each is grateful for the life still possible. They have decades of rich memories to share that Laura often fondly recalls for them to talk about. And, most especially, they have the love of their adult children and grandchildren.

What helps Laura most is her support system. As they have done for many years, she and a group of five other women meet for two hours every Wednesday morning. Calling themselves "Sip and Giggle," they talk over coffee and find humor as well as valuable insight in sharing the concerns they have in common. All are about the same age, so have similar losses and worries for their loved ones' health. Laura is uplifted by long visits (mostly by telephone) shared with a "kind and helpful" daughter who lives nearby. In addition, for the past 20 years, Laura and four girlfriends, who have stayed in touch since childhood, meet for five days every year in a different city. Their nickname is the "Warwick Waddlers." They all grew up on Warwick Lane in a suburb of St. Louis, "and by now, we all waddle," Laura lightheartedly explains. "There is always much laughter and sharing," she says.

Laura also deals with stress by staying active. She volunteers twice a month at a shelter for homeless people and twice monthly helps cook for another organization that feeds hungry people in a different part of town. She volunteers to help out at church-related events, too. For exercise, she keeps trying to get into a regular routine of taking 30-minute walks on their treadmill or in the backyard.

Laura knows the wisdom of focusing on what her husband can still do and the life they can enjoy together. At least for now, they can continue living in their own home. She also knows and can remind Mark of his legacy. Throughout his ministry, he was decades ahead of most Americans in his work for equal rights for women, African Americans, and others who were and still are marginalized, including mentally ill and poor people. His impassioned published articles on social justice issues went out to 50,000 readers in the journal he edited, and as a pastor he also touched the lives of countless appreciative parishioners, the couples he counseled and married, and the dozens of young ministers he mentored. He is a man whose life was lived for others and who needs to be reminded that he is widely respected and deeply loved.[5]

CARING FOR A PARENT

There is a delicate balance to be maintained as our caregiving increases. Even when we are genuinely glad to give back caring that was given to us, something highly valuable is lost when we experience a fragile parent who must rely on us for kindness and to be kept safe. It *is* an emotional jolt, a shocker, when we're absolutely forced to be the grown-up in the room. Except for carrying within ourselves the positive and negative life lessons our parents have left us with, we are now the decision makers responsible for stabilizing their and our universe. Our parent's dignity and personhood as an adult seems diminished, and we want to protect it.

Baltimore physician Cecilia Brennecke, writing about visiting her 90-year-old mother in a Minnesota assisted living facility, describes one of the most painful parts of grieving the loss of one's parent before she dies. As the months between visits pass, Dr. Brennecke sees that her mother's memory is worse every time she visits, yet she is comforted by the realization that her mother "has never yet failed to recognize me, although recognition has been a little slow lately." Fortunately, "she smiles and greets me by name, introduces me all around with all three names, first, middle and nickname. Names she gave me. Relief floods over me each time." But later on, leaving her mother's room, writes Dr. Brennecke, "I overhear [a] fellow patient ask who I am. I almost cry when I hear the answer." She is "some lady from church," her mother says.[6]

Such gut-wrenching experiences probably signal our need not to swallow the pain but to allow ourselves those solemn tears. Remembering all that our parent was able to give us, before this advanced dementia changed everything, is painful. On the other side of that pain, however, is gratitude. Even if sometimes we're afraid to let ourselves fully feel the sadness, for fear it will overwhelm us, crying is part of healing. Expressing our feelings to a friend or writing in a journal helps us move forward.

Remember that you are strong. Working through the stages of mourning is necessary, but your feelings will not take control of you. Allowing the emotions of sorrow, regret, guilt, and anger to be expressed will enable your sweet memories to flow. There is much to be thankful for, we realize, as our grief and healing process progress.

As the late psychologist and bereavement expert John Schneider once said, "I have to know what I've lost to know what I have left, what is still possible."[7] Most of us can see in ourselves certain positive character traits and values that came from our parents. We can call to mind valuable lessons learned and precious memories from the decades that went before. We can recall who our parents were and their strengths that prevailed for most of those long years lived.

Dr. Brennecke remembers her mother as a "teacher, a mother of eight [married for 65 years], with an adoring husband . . . [a woman who] could grow anything, could sew beautifully, always dressed impeccably and didn't care for entertaining."[8] Most surely, she can bring to mind the various ways her mother played a large role in raising a daughter with the wherewithal to work hard and become an accomplished, highly respected medical director of radiology for Johns Hopkins.

BLESSINGS, SORROWS, AND AXES TO GRIND

Grief is complicated and conflict ridden because human feelings and relationships are so complicated. Whether our childhood or overall relationship with our now impaired elderly parent was very good, good, reasonably all right, awful, or abusive—there remains a young part of us (which psychologists call our "inner child") that is still coping with and trying to figure out our parents. Even after we've loved and been a caregiver to our own children or nieces and nephews and watched them grow into adulthood, still a young part of us seeks parental approval.

What is it my parent expects of me? What did my mother or father always say about growing old or disabled or dying? What promises did I make regarding their elder care, either to myself or to them? Whether we are religious or not, "Honor thy Mother and Father" is a commandment deeply embedded in our individual value systems.

If our parent wasn't able to be the good mother or father we needed—because of their own deprivations in childhood, character flaws, afflictions, addictions, workaholic tendencies, or the like—most of us still wanted their approval and love. Part of grieving that frail elderly parent's mental deterioration is facing the fact that any chance of reconciliation or a loving final chapter is forever gone. Although those windows and doors of opportunity for having a different relationship with that parent probably closed a long time ago, dementia locks up the house.

Thus, whether our parent left us with a rich and meaningful connection to him or her and wonderful memories or an utter lack of fulfillment of that yearning for a loving parent, it is painful to watch our parent cease to be the person we gratefully loved or hoped would someday do a better job of loving us.

Like most of you who are reading this book, my own parents gave me a mixture of blessings to cherish, sorrows to mourn, and axes to grind. How each of them moved into old age is an entirely different story.

My mother's dementia was longer in unfolding and worse in how debilitating it became, yet Mama was the easier one to care for because she remained appreciative of the things we did for her. She showed such humble gratitude when I would give her a manicure and pedicure and trim the little hairs from her chin. Night after night, she ate slowly and truly *cherished* the McDonald's burgers and fries that she and my dad almost always wanted for supper. But, as the Alzheimer's disease worsened, Mama was hospitalized with pneumonia and other medical problems from which we were told she would not recover. Our mother was a loving person with a deep faith and trust in God, but we saw that she was suffering physically, emotionally, and spiritually because she couldn't grasp what was going on. After she'd ripped the miserably uncomfortable respirator out of her throat, asking aloud why God was making her suffer, my siblings and I agreed not to have the doctors reinsert the respirator. We decided that the most merciful thing was to have our mother moved into hospice care, with only the little nose-piece device giving her oxygen. We were blessed to have several days with her before she died.

Our dad lived to be 96 by comparison to our mother's 89 years. He stayed mentally healthy and physically active longer (conducting farm business, making financial decisions, and admirably walking several miles a day into his 80s). Yet it was our dad who was the huge challenge to deal with—even without dementia—as he was the one who never said thank you, was demanding, and was often unkind in how he spoke to our mother. As he became more physically frail and emotionally vulnerable, we also saw that he was in danger of being manipulated into *literally* giving away the family farm (to a so-called good neighbor lady, solicitous with flattery even in the presence of our mother).

My siblings had long tried to persuade our parents to move near my sister to improve the quality of their lives. Along with living in a state distant from all three of us, each had frailties that made them awfully vulnerable. We wanted our folks to be safe from being mistreated or otherwise preyed upon by anyone, especially caregivers. Finally they agreed, sold their home, and moved to a new house in Texas. There my sister and brother were generous in providing care, supervised a daytime paid companion, arranged for Meals on Wheels, and saw to it that one of us siblings was always available at night.

During my visits home when my mother was still alive, I was glad to run errands and do yard work, just to get out of the house and not have to hear my father speak unkindly about someone in the family or tell another story for the hundredth time. After our dad was a widower and bedridden, my siblings and I never confronted him on how, for years on end, he too often had spoken disrespectfully and hurtfully to our mother, and routinely had my brother, my sister, or me in the "dog house" for imagined wrongs.

When he was no longer powerful but dependent on our care, it was sad to see him so frail. When each of us siblings visited, we sat for hours by his bed, watched televised college football games or reruns of *The Lawrence Welk Show* that he and our mother had watched decades ago, and listened while he talked. It was the right thing to do. Our mother had loved him, and they were married for 71 years. I loved him, too. He was an honest, decent man, a good provider, and as good a grandfather and father as he knew how to be.

But my dad was often critical and almost impossible to please. Even as adults my siblings and I had to deal with his demands. When I was a 55-year-old college professor and visited them in Oklahoma, my dad expected me to go with him to the family farm to do work that seemed to me pointless: while he gave orders and watched, I cut down trees where no crops were going to be planted anyway. And even during the hottest part of a 100-degree summer day, our dad would insist that my older brother dig through rock-hard ground to remove some half-buried stones from their backyard. He expected the two of us to work like the farmhands we used to be while our sister was expected to drive 200 miles to take him to a doctor's appointment. We all three acquired a good, strong work ethic from our parents, but from our dad we learned to overwork at our own expense.

My siblings and I did what our dad told us to do. We did it because we knew he expected it, and because not to do what he asked would upset our mother and say to both of our parents that we didn't love and respect them. This wasn't just about "honoring" our father; we were behaving as we'd learned to behave from our mother, who cherished my dad all her life. *Sometimes as adults, we just have to accept our parents as the people they are and trust that they did the best that they could. We ourselves have to grow strong, forgive ourselves when we aren't as strong as we think we ought to be, and figure out how to do the best that we can— in exasperating situations—to interact kindly with our parent(s).*

Despite my own work to become more compassionate toward my father, I still had plenty of moments when the old anger surfaced. Our hearts, minds, and emotions are not always perfectly aligned, and that's okay. I write about my own struggle not to make this appear easy but to affirm that it is hard, imperfect work that nevertheless has its rewards.

All human relationships are complicated in one way or another or in many ways. Being intimidated by or feeling resentful of a parent doesn't mean that you don't love them or aren't grateful as their daughter or son. Having mixed feelings about the people we care about isn't being disloyal, it's just being human. Yet it is the task of every mature, moral adult to accept the responsibility for making our own lives into something good and to move beyond blaming others. *It's up to each of us to find the best life within reach.*

Especially important is remembering that our parents could only do the best they knew to do at the time. In raising us, they coped as well as they could then. Part of the grieving process of watching our parents in their frail elder years involves making our peace with whatever went wrong in the family or families where we grew up. As someone once said, "Holding on to bitterness is like taking poison and waiting for the other person to die."[9] We have to acknowledge and then let go of old anger, regrets, and encumbrances of all kinds as adult children. Grievances need to be worked through and released. For those of you who suffered profound abuse—more than having to deal with a critical, cranky, or overly demanding parent—working through grievances is a task of a higher order.

Sometimes old hurts and axes to grind necessitate our going to see a psychologist, counselor, social worker, or clergy person for help. You can measure the degree of your own health and your fitness to be a responsible caregiver by honestly asking yourself whether you are a kind person with empathy toward the impaired elder in your care and others who are vulnerable. If your present relationships are healthy, mostly working well and loving, you probably have made peace with your past.

A WORD OF CAUTION

But making peace with your past can be hard work. It is especially difficult if you are a son, daughter, or sibling who was severely abused or neglected as a child; if you have been a victim of spousal abuse; or if you have an alcohol or other substance abuse problem. If so, you are at risk of being a neglectful or an *abusive* caretaker. Likewise, if you struggle with impatience and say demeaning things to your dependent family member or in other ways have trouble controlling your anger, it is urgent that you get support from others. Please seek the professional help you need for their protection, your own healing, and to keep yourself out of prison. Other family members or paid caretakers need to be in charge of providing the needed safe and compassionate care.

SEEING THE BIG PICTURE

As much as ingratitude is unattractive at any age, so is rigidity. It's different when someone has dementia and is obsessed with wearing the same pair of worn-out and raggedy slacks. That person might have loved a closetful of different outfits until her brain disease dramatically changed her personality, through no fault or control of her own. By contrast, for as long as you can remember, maybe one of your parents would get an idea that something should be done a certain way and hold on to it like a dog with a bone. And if one of your mom or dad's failings included not seeming to notice how other people felt, it can help you to consider what you know about your parent's childhood. Sensitivity to others' feelings may not have been part of the family's playbook. Was being tough—in order to survive hardships—valued and expected, instead of tenderness?

What I hope to practice, as a lesson well learned from not wanting to be lacking in empathy like some people I've known, is the attitude of thoughtfulness that my mother exemplified. I want to be able to "hear" what other people are feeling and be a compassionate person.

In the words of my closest and longtime friend, Marian, "As I age, I want to be mindful that the world is not just about me." Throughout their lives, our mothers had kind hearts. Even with advanced dementia, Marian's mother and my own were mindful of their caregivers and generous in showing appreciation.

It is a necessary part of mental health and maturity to see the whole picture. Although recognizing ways that my dad was not the parent I wished he could have been, I remember having many good times with the man I called "Daddy," whose nicknames for me were "Sidekick" and "Partner." When I was a tomboy/cowgirl always ready to ride with him to the John Deere store, I loved so many things about working outdoors, feeding farm animals, and riding my horse across the pasture to bring in the milk cow. Most of all, I'm glad that my dad, as a granddad, enjoyed and was loving toward my daughters, both as children and as young adults.

Absolutely everyone's parents had failings. Our own children must cope with the various ways we've taken their strengths and good deeds for granted, had skin too thin and reacted in anger to something said innocently or left unsaid, been judgmental or insistent on having things our way. We are all guilty of being poor role models, some of the time or often, making unwise decisions or behaving selfishly.

What will prepare us for the future is to recognize the strengths our parents had and the valuable lessons they've provided, even if our parents had a bevy of failings. If we are honest with ourselves, we have traits of good character and other personal qualities worth nurturing that we gained during our growing-up years. We hope our own children will be similarly kind in getting beyond *our* faults to affirm and emulate our better selves.

In my mother, I saw an inner strength and spiritual life that enabled her to hold her head high and remain a sweet, loving person, even when dealing with my father caused her pain. From Mama, I also learned to notice and deeply appreciate small acts of kindness. I saw that it's always important to set aside money for people who need it more than you. I learned to love fresh flowers and ice cream and cook amazing pumpkin pies. I learned to keep trying to become a better person, with an ever-more-thankful heart. From this forgiving, caring, soft-spoken Mama, I learned to believe in a God who loves unconditionally because that's how she loved all of us.

From my dad, I learned about more than work. I learned to love sports, dogs, horses, wheat fields and pastures, wide open spaces and long walks. From him, I learned that music, dancing, and exercise are good for the soul and are three of the best possible ways to relieve stress and enjoy life. Yes, dancing. My farmer father liked to dance my mother around the living room. For hours at a time, for as long as he lived, daddy played or had someone play for him a huge stack of CDs with lively country, folk, and polka music. I also learned that some lucky people could live to be 96 and still smoke cigars like a chimney.

For those of us fortunate enough to have had grandparents active in our lives, there is more to be learned. From my Granny I learned that the keys to a life well-lived are to avoid self-pity, keep reading and learning, remain open to new experiences and opportunities to travel, enjoy chocolate and root beer floats as often as possible, and keep a sense of humor. My Granny lost her father and mother young, was sexually abused by a stepfather, finished growing up in an orphanage, never went to school past the eighth grade, worked as a maid for a rich woman, then (the day after she married at 18) traveled with my grandfather to homestead in the Oklahoma Territory just after statehood.

From more than 30 years of studying resilient people, I see that my Granny did what hardy people often do: she learned from harsh life experiences, refused to remain bitter over the great losses and abuse she suffered as a young person, stayed open to adventure and new perspectives, always kept looking for ways to help other people, and had a strong network of social support from family, friends, her garden club, and her church.

As a widow, Granny took a college course to learn how to write short stories. This was at the age of 69, living with me when I was a college freshman. At 75, she traveled and stayed with me again while I studied in Scotland for a year. We lived in one large room with twin beds and shared a (mostly) cold-water bathroom and tiny kitchen with half a dozen other people. In her 70s and early 80s, Granny regularly visited the folks she called "the old people" at the local nursing home and died there herself at the age of 89.

I hope to be just like my Granny in as many ways possible. She was generous in writing letters and sending cards to her children and grandchildren, and generous with the checks she enclosed when $25 or $35 felt to a young person like $200 would feel today.

She was remarkably nonjudgmental for a person who was born in 1891 and deeply religious. She never spoke about my smoking cigarettes in those years of college, graduate school, and later, or commented on my pierced ears (both of which I knew she rather associated with "loose" women). Like my mother's love, Granny's love was unconditional. I love my own daughters the same way.

MIXED LESSONS FROM OUR ELDERS ON GROWING OLD

It is a theme I will return to in this book, again and again: What kind of an elderly person will I / will you become? God willing, luck prevailing, or with good health habits and despite bad habits, if our fate is to live long lives, what lessons do we need to take from our parents, grandparents, aunts and uncles, older siblings, and others if our goal is to follow their good example or avoid the negative ways they lived in old age?

FEW REGRETS

Ruth Marian Misemer was a woman who knew that she didn't want her loved ones to be burdened with regret whenever it came time for her to die. "If something happens to me," she would say to her adult children, Marian and David, at the end of holiday visits, "I don't want you to feel bad because I've had a good life. I've loved my life and I will be okay."

Especially when Mrs. Misemer began a long journey with Alzheimer's disease, these were comforting words that resonated with her children and their families. Because of the quality and fullness of the life their beloved mother and grandmother already had lived, she was an inspiration to everyone. All of the family members were strengthened by her love for them and theirs for her, even while grieving her gradual slipping away from herself and from them.

Regret is one of the hardest emotions to deal with when losing someone you love, whether from death, estrangement, or the ravages of dementia. We mourn what was done that cannot be undone, relationships that were torn apart but never healed, and our loved one's unfulfilled dreams or unachieved desire to have left the world or others' lives in a better place.

In the four decades I've been teaching grief counseling to physicians and other medical professionals, funeral directors, counselors, and clergy, I've often been asked whether regret is the stage in a mourning process where people most often get stuck. Yes, it is. Along with anger, guilt, and depression, sorrowfully wishing that our own or a loved one's life had been lived in ways very different—when it's too late to change—is a reality terribly painful for most people.

Although Mrs. Misemer never got the education that she dreamed of as a young woman nor was able to use her beautiful voice to sing professionally, a dream of her girlhood, Mrs. Misemer was thankful for, felt fulfilled by, and was at peace with her life. And she shared those feelings with her family. She took a quiet pride in having made a home for her family in many communities in eight different states, as a result of frequent moves due to her husband's work. Although each move was a challenge, she approached it with a determination to make an adventure of it, volunteered at the kids' schools, always joined the church choir, and helped out in activities such as the Boy Scouts. She was loved for her kindness, gentle spirit, sense of fun, and her beautiful singing voice.

Mrs. Misemer was said to "wear her faith lightly," meaning she didn't take her beliefs lightly but she respected others' beliefs, having known so many people of different religions and ethnic backgrounds from all those years of moving around the country. She was forgiving of people, and, even after Alzheimer's disease robbed her of more nuanced thinking, she would say of someone who was rude or unkind, "Oh, he probably ate something that disagreed with him!"

It is well known that when other kinds of knowledge and memory are lost, music is often one of the last things to be taken away by Alzheimer's disease. When she could no longer prepare one of her delicious meals, take care of her home, or write the notes her family and friends treasured, Mrs. Misemer could still play the piano and sing the hymns she had loved for a lifetime. When she could no longer sing the words, she could still hum the melodies to favorite songs, continuing to share music with those around her in the memory care unit where her life ended.

What lessons can be taken from Mrs. Misemer's life, applicable to our own inevitable aging, regardless of how "well" we grow old or whether someday we have our own battle with dementia? The answer is that we will have done an enduring good deed if, from observing what our parents did well or poorly, we can spare our spouses, siblings, children, and grandchildren from having to regret the way we lived our lives.

We can pass on the gift of overcoming our disappointments and transcending our losses or tragedies, to leave behind a life well lived. In this way our loved ones, who will care for us when *we* are frail elders and survive us at death, can mourn with sadness for themselves but mostly not for us.

"TUNING UP" FOR OLD AGE

What did *you* learn from your parents and grandparents? Have you thought about how one becomes an elderly person of the kind caregivers are glad to care for?

For certain, as I see it, we don't suddenly become grateful or unselfish in late adulthood. At every age, we can benefit from expanding our personalities to become more patient, less demanding, and much more appreciative of the things others do for us. We will be happier and our loved ones will find it more rewarding to spend time with us if "thank you" are the words we say genuinely and most often.

Of course, some things are beyond our control. Like the impact of Reverend Mark's head injuries, some conditions can render an elderly person's brain less able to control the expression of gruffness or critical comments. However, absent neurological damage that may change our personalities in some negative ways, we can practice positive attitudes and behaviors *now* as a "tune-up" for when our family members or paid caregivers will be looking after us.

"HAPPINESS IS A CHOICE"

In a provocative program produced for public television, *The Happiness Advantage*, Shawn Achor tells how *habits* "can rewire the brain for higher levels of optimism." Drawing upon "more than a decade of teaching and researching positive psychology at Harvard University," Achor explains "why happiness is a choice, and how . . . a whopping 90 percent of [our] happiness is based on how [we] process the world."[10]

Achor is a young researcher with the wisdom of a sage when he says, "Change the lens through which you view the world and reap the happiness advantage." One of his suggestions for becoming a more hopeful, life-affirming person is called "The Three Gratitudes." For 21 days in a row—the time Achor says is needed to create a new life habit—"write down and say out loud three things you're grateful for and why, specifically over the last 24 hours, and never repeat the same gratitude over the 21 days."[11]

For example, when I write in my own gratitude journal, which I keep by my bedside table, I number each gratitude and write complete sentences in which I avoid generalities and name specifics that fit the present: (1) I'm thankful that my daughter Amanda had a Slurpee waiting for me after my dental surgery today. (2) I'm thankful that my daughter Ashley invited me to dinner at her place tomorrow night so I can see the new paint job she just finished in the bathroom. (3) I'm thankful that Panda, our border collie, is feeling better today after getting her vaccinations yesterday.

Having to name three different things each day and not repeat a gratitude for 21 days requires that we notice and name many things that we might not stop to notice and be thankful for. As the exercise continues, studies show that others begin to see us as being "more attractive" and "optimistic" and are more likely to enjoy spending time with us. After all, who doesn't want to be with a positive person more than a complainer who is always seeing the glass half empty? We feel happier because we are becoming more mindful of what is good in life. Others are apt to find our increased optimism contagious.

Achor's "Charge Your Battery" habit-changing exercise offers another valuable way to grow, for those of us wanting to be more kindhearted as caregivers and hoping to thrive in our own elder years when needing help. "The greatest predictor of happiness and health," says Achor, is "having meaningful social connections." For 21 days in a row, this exercise involves writing a positive note or an e-mail offering someone a word of "praise or thanksgiving, 21 different people in 21 days."[12]

It's important, Achor cautions, to do these 21-day habit-changing exercises one at a time. His research shows that trying to make too many changes at once often results in feeling frustrated and giving up on trying to instill new ways of viewing the world.

You may think that you don't *know* 21 different people to thank. But consider the broad array of folks with whom you've come in contact, in one way or another, over the years and more recently. Worth remembering with a word of thanks are former classmates or teachers, or a coach or Scout leader who made an impact on you or one of your children. Deserving of a note of appreciation might be a neighbor, physician, nurse, your rabbi, priest, or minister. Or, perhaps, an e-mail to a niece, nephew, or other relative whose visit or correspondence came at a fortunate time. You can write something in a card to the mechanic who keeps your car running well or the volunteer who provides a service or a paid caregiver who has done something thoughtful for your elderly loved one. And no one likes receiving an actual letter in the mail more than your young grandchild who delights you with the drawings she makes in school, in order to "make happy" your refrigerator door.

Giving others a genuine word of praise or thanks—in a note, card, or e-mail, day after day, a different person for three weeks—is a simple but very effective way to become happier and more gracious in our human relationships. Not only will you brighten the days of each of the recipients of your words of appreciation, you will also be energized; as Achor puts it, you will "charge your [own] battery." With 21 days of this exercise and another 21 days with the gratitude exercise, we can put ourselves on a path to grow in optimism. We can nurture these new habits that change the lens through which we see the world, making us less likely to feel depressed under the stress of being caregivers.

DRAWING STRENGTH FROM NATURE'S BEAUTY

One of the most nurturing and healing things you can do for yourself and for your impaired elderly loved one, is to sit outdoors in the sun—alone or together—or take a drive where there are trees, green or freshly plowed fields, rolling hills or farm animals grazing, vineyards or rock formations, bodies of water, interesting bridges, or awesome skies. Experiences of beauty are available to all of us to draw upon for comfort, inspiration, and strength. From what is lovely in nature, a sense of gratitude also can be deeply felt.

As I write this, it just stopped raining a few minutes ago, in the suburban part of Baltimore where I live. I felt compelled to jump up from my desk and run around to the front yard of our house to look east, in search of a rainbow. It has been a gorgeous fall day and still is. I've seen rainbows many times in conditions like these, when the rain subsides and the sun is lowering in the west. But there is no multicolored arch in the sky today.

What I *can* see are the colors red, yellow, orange, and khaki decorating the trees in every direction, leaves still clinging to their broad branches, colorfully aglow in mid-October. The sky is also spectacular everywhere I look: shades of blue, pink, and purple behind beautifully majestic white and gray billowing clouds.

And suddenly I am thinking of my parents. From their hilltop gravesite, overlooking a seemingly endless western Oklahoma horizon, I've counted 71 proud tall turbines in the surrounding sea of wind farms. My love of the sky is a gift from my parents and a gift from growing up in rural Oklahoma. There our sky was wide open, always interesting, often as blue as the Gulf of Mexico or as white as the Rocky Mountain peaks in winter, strikingly pretty and in every season spaciously grand.

My mother found strength in looking to the nighttime sky. Where we lived, no city lights dimmed the brightness of the night, and she never failed to call our attention to the Milky Way, the Big Dipper and other constellations, and every falling star. As a farmer, my dad was always watching the weather in the daytime sky, tracking cloud formations that signaled calm or an approaching storm. He seemed to draw a sense of peace just from long periods of sky watching and also from sitting in his Chevy pickup on a hill overlooking our wheat field, where sometimes I sat with him, watching the wheat grow.

When both of my parents were frail and near the end of their lives, they still wanted to sit outdoors for long periods, as they always had done, whether wrapped in winter's heavy jackets and a blanket apiece or in the short sleeves of spring, summer, and fall. Even in their tiny yard, clearly it continued to comfort them to watch the changing cloud formations in the sky. The calm they experienced was palpable to any observer, as my folks breathed in the fresh air, watched birds alight on fence posts and squirrels scamper about near their feet. Sitting there with my parents and sometimes alone gave sustenance to my soul as well.

Whatever else I have gained from being my parents' younger daughter, I learned to love nature's beauty and weather watching, in all seasons, through forecasts bad and good. From them I learned to notice and be grateful for "all creatures great and small." Today I am grateful for these memories and for the pleasure and sense of empowerment that I still receive from enjoying nature and watching the sky.

I believe it will enrich your life, too, never to let a day or a night go by without looking up to explore, experience, and cherish the clouds or stars or blue sky overhead. There is strength to be drawn from so much that is worthy of notice in nature's power and beauty, even from indoors when it's rainy or blustery or cold.

Depending on where you grew up, there may be other parts of nature beyond what I have just described, experiences of beauty that your parents shared with you, that can help you gain a sense of renewal, hope, or strength.

Caregiving can be richly rewarding but it is also extremely stressful. There are many ways to draw upon the natural world for sustenance. All we have to do is open our eyes.

Is This Normal Aging
or Dementia?

Even more epidemic than Alzheimer's itself is the fear of Alzheimer's.
—Richard Lipton, MD, Albert Einstein College of Medicine

When it comes to considering our fate in the near or not-so-distant future, there is probably nothing more disturbing that having one of these thoughts: Are *my* occasional memory problems the beginning of dementia? What will be *my* fate in old age? How long will *I* be able to live on my own? Have I / have we saved enough money for the years ahead? Who will take care of me or us? Will *my* children put *me* in a nursing home?

While caring for an elderly family member, we are likely to worry at times about our own as well as our loved one's memory lapses, slowed decision making, and any physical or mental impairments. Even in our 50s and especially in our 60s or 70s, it is normal for each of us to feel some anxiety about our own aging brain. Such concerns often skyrocket as we watch a loved one's brain functioning go from good to somewhat bad to sadly much worse.

Stressed, we may wonder what course our loved one's aging will take, and what course our own aging will take. Often, in the last few years of my mother's life and after her death at age 89, I wondered whether my aging would mirror hers. Would I become increasingly frail? Would I suffer from Alzheimer's at the end? Confronting my own inevitable process of aging, I asked myself was there anything—*is there anything*—I can control?

Fortunately, the research completed for this book has confirmed what I had already learned as a psychologist over the years: Except in rather rare cases, we are not simply at the mercy of our genes. There are no guarantees for any of us as individuals, of course, but a broad range of studies show that wise lifestyle choices and the prevention or early treatment of certain health problems can significantly reduce our risk factors for dementia or delay its onset. "Aging successfully" is something all of us want for ourselves and, to the greatest extent possible, we want the same for our physically or cognitively impaired loved one.

If you have anxious moments when your mind seems to go blank and you suddenly can't remember the name of a person you know well, can't recall the name of a movie star in a film you saw a few days ago or whether on this particular day you've taken a certain medication, I hope to ease your mind. One of my goals in this chapter is to provide enough detailed information that you can distinguish between changed behaviors and problems with remembering things that are worth worrying about and those that are most likely simply part of a normal aging process so that you can see when a complete medical evaluation is needed.

The good news is that the odds of having dementia—also called major neurocognitive disorder (NCD)—are just "1%–2% at age 65 and [I have to add the word *only* here!] as high as 30% by age 85."[1] While mild neurocognitive problems are considerably more common, you do not have to worry when you sometimes have trouble remembering a name. Many young people say they are "terrible at remembering names," and almost everyone who is good at it uses the word association or other memory strategies that become more necessary as we grow older.

In my earlier years as a college professor, I learned nearly all 150 to 200 of my students' names during the first week of classes, every semester. These days (10,000 students later), it takes me three or four weeks to memorize the names that go with those bright young faces, a task that now requires a seating chart plus a lot of conscious effort and name repetition. As long as our brains remain healthy, we continue to learn in our 60s and beyond, just more slowly and strategically.

NORMAL AGING

As my good friend Blake Wattenbarger, a human factors psychologist, explains, "With aging, the main effect on cognition is that thinking slows down. For complex reasoning tasks, requiring holding lots of information in short term memory, the slowness of thinking can prevent getting to the end of a long chain of reasoning before short term memory fails, so reasoning itself seems to be failing, when it is only slowing down. I've wondered if this accounts for the common observation that mathematicians mostly make their best contributions by age 30, and are pretty much useless after age 50."[2]

Generally speaking, yes, it is true that the ability to speedily process or analyze new information slows down steadily from the 20s to the late 80s. Also true is the fact that in virtually every culture (worldwide), wisdom is associated with growing old.

As we age, we continue to exercise good judgment, comprehend words, and benefit from our accumulated experience and knowledge. It should tell us something about the ongoing competency of the aging brain that *all* of the justices of the Supreme Court of the United States of America are old enough for senior citizen discounts and AARP membership.

Hearing losses rise increasingly for many people at ages 65 to 74 and sharply rise from ages 75 to 85 and beyond (more so in men). Vision impairments rise steadily from ages 65 to 85 and older (more so in women).[3] For these reasons and because we absorb new knowledge more deliberately, asking someone to speak more slowly or repeat what was said or needing more time to read something before mastering it and giving a response is a normal part of the aging process for many men and women.

Recalling well-learned general information much more readily than the details or order of occurrence of everyday experiences is a common experience. Needing to concentrate more intently and with fewer distractions when learning new information, multitasking, driving in heavy traffic to an unfamiliar location, or when taking a different route is normal, too.

Finding it harder to remember which friend said a certain thing or to which adult child something was said is just part of accumulating so many different experiences in life, just as it's hard to remember whether you've locked the door to your car when you've done it countless *thousands* of times by the age of 60 or so.

Forgetting an appointment, name, place, event, or word and recalling it a few minutes, hours, or even a day later is understandable for the same reason as mentioned above. Reminders and various memory strategies are helpful when we are young; more such reminders are helpful and often necessary as we grow older.

Walking from the kitchen to the bedroom for an item, forgetting what you went after, returning to the kitchen, then remembering it is usually a function of not concentrating or having many things on one's mind at once. This happens to almost everyone but more often in our senior years.

I also want to emphasize just how much the high stress of caregiving can leave a person frazzled, emotionally drained, and pulled in multiple directions, preoccupied with so many responsibilities that one's concentration is impaired, making the caregiver at times quite absentminded or forgetful.

CHERRY MARQUEZ

My friend Cherry is a terrific example of a woman in her 60s whose brain worked perfectly fine most of the time, yet she had some alarming memory lapses as a caregiver overloaded with stress. One such experience of dangerous distraction and forgetting almost led to burning down her home!

Cherry Marquez dearly loved her mother-in-law, who lived in a nearby apartment, was a widow, nearly blind, and was dependent on Cherry for almost everything except for bathing and dressing herself. Cherry took the elderly woman grocery shopping, to church, and to doctor's appointments. She did her mother in law's housekeeping, laundry, and meal preparation. At the same time, although Cherry had retired from an accomplished career as a first-grade teacher, she was still very busy babysitting her grandson and helping out a recently divorced daughter.

Cherry's mother-in-law never had much of an appetite but *loved* hard-boiled eggs. So Cherry would cook a potful and take the elderly woman 8 to 10 of the already cooked eggs every week. With so many caregiving jobs as a wife, daughter-in-law, grandmother, and mother simultaneously on her mind, Cherry thought she had gotten multitasking down to a science. "Not so fast," she later reminded herself. Having too much on her mind had led to several close calls while driving distracted and to a nearly disastrous accident at home.

On an afternoon when a reception was to be held, with the mayor of Denver present, honoring her younger daughter's achievements, Cherry was (as usual) trying to do several things at once before hopping in the car for the 40-minute drive to Denver. One of those things, Cherry told me, was "boiling eggs for Grandma."

It was a lovely celebratory event. Cherry and her husband, Lorenzo, and their elder daughter, Monica, were so proud of Christine's leadership of Me Casa, a nonprofit group that works with Hispanic families for outreach. It was a joy to see Christine so happy, her hard work and dedication appreciated.

As Cherry and her husband drove back home in their separate cars—four or five hours after Cherry placed nearly a dozen eggs in a pan on the stove—Cherry remembered! All she could think of was the fire trucks she expected to see in front of their house. Thankfully, she thought to herself, at least she'd be arriving home ahead of Lorenzo.

There were no fire trucks! Running into the house, however, Cherry was met with a foul odor. There she encountered a kitchen with eggs that had exploded everywhere—all over the ceiling, walls, curtains, and floor. On the flat-top electric stove was a pan red-hot on the bottom and otherwise completely black. She put the pan in the sink and ran to the garage. "Lorenzo," she exclaimed, "please don't go in! I have to tell you what I've done!"

"It was a huge mess," Cherry told me, "but he never said a word. We worked for two hours cleaning it up until I said, 'Please, Lorenzo, please go on to bed.' I needed to finish cleaning it up because it was totally my fault. I got up on a ladder to clean the ceiling, went to bed at midnight, and said a prayer: 'Thank you, God, that I didn't set our house on fire!'"

Looking back, Cherry says, "For days after, while cleaning splattered boiled eggs from the ceiling, I repeated that prayer." Early on, she carried the vivid memory of how scared she had been and simply felt relieved. But then it became a funny story, told again and again to family and friends. "So many times, one of the things that gets you through is humor, and sometimes self-deprecating humor," Cherry recalled. "You just had to die laughing!"

MAJOR CONFUSION AND BEHAVIORAL CHANGE

An episode of being accident prone under stress or struggling to recall a name is a normal part of aging, even if occasionally you have the alarming experience of "blanking" on the name of someone like your longtime neighbor, LaKeita, whose name comes to mind soon thereafter or later in the day. When you should worry about your brain health or your elderly loved one's cognitive decline is when *who LaKeita is*—is not remembered *at all*.

It might also set off a useful internal alarm system if you notice that your spouse, parent, grandparent, or sibling is repeatedly showing confusion in a way that is completely out of character, such as laboring to complete a familiar task (operate the microwave, find the exit door at the grocery store, address a greeting card, or balance a checkbook) when that task used to be no problem at all. In such a situation, it *is* important to ask yourself and your family doctor whether this changed behavior is just normal aging—perhaps the result of fatigue and stress or the side effect of medications, something temporary that can be remedied—or something requiring a more extensive medical evaluation. Your loved one's physician will do a thorough physical exam and will probably order some tests to help determine whether these problems are the result of a reversible cause (examples include depression, a thyroid problem, an infection, or vitamin B12 deficiency) or due to a progressive illness only somewhat treatable such as Alzheimer's disease, something causing cognitive impairments that are gradually getting worse.

HARRY'S STORY

Cognitive changes can sneak up, but new behaviors can in fact be red flags, especially if they are repeated and come to be a new pattern. A man who would later be diagnosed with a type of Alzheimer's disease showed behavioral changes that *should* raise a red flag. In *Fundamentals of Abnormal Psychology*, the textbook I use in one of the courses I teach, author Ronald Comer draws from a case study by psychiatrist Leonard Heston:

> Harry appeared to be in perfect health at age 58 . . . He worked in the municipal water treatment plant of a small city, and it was at work that the first overt signs of Harry's mental illness appeared. While responding to a minor emergency, he became confused about the correct order in which to pull the levers that controlled the flow of fluids. As a result, several thousand gallons of raw sewage were discharged into a river. Harry had been an efficient and diligent worker, so after puzzled questioning, his error was attributed to the flu and overlooked.
>
> Several weeks later, Harry came home with a baking dish his wife had asked him to buy, having forgotten that he had brought home the identical dish two nights before. Later that week, on two successive nights, he went to pick up his daughter at her job at her restaurant, apparently forgetting that she had changed shifts and was now working days. A month after that, he quite uncharacteristically argued with . . . the phone company; he was trying to pay a bill that he had already paid three days before.
>
> Months passed and Harry's wife was beside herself. She could see that his problem was worsening. Not only had she been unable to get effective help, but Harry himself was becoming resentful and sometimes suspicious

of her attempts. He now insisted there was nothing wrong with him, and she would catch him narrowly watching her every movement . . . Sometimes he became angry—sudden little storms without apparent cause . . . More difficult for his wife was Harry's repetitiveness in conversation: He often repeated stories from the past and sometimes repeated isolated phrases and sentences from more recent exchanges. There was no content and little continuity in his choice of subjects.[4]

This is an unusual case. Harry suffered from a rare major neurocognitive disorder that typically strikes at a younger age and progresses at a faster pace than most all but the (also less common) early-onset type of Alzheimer's. His case illustrates how problems at work and other lapses viewed in hindsight make it clear that something was seriously wrong. Since accidents can happen to anyone and he was a good worker, the early signs weren't recognized as such when Harry failed to perform an on-the-job task that he'd done correctly probably hundreds of times.

"Two years after Harry had first allowed the sewage to escape, he was clearly a changed man," explains Dr. Heston. "Most of the time he seemed preoccupied; he usually had a vacant smile on his face, and what little he said was so vague that it lacked meaning."[5] Harry's wife became his everyday caregiver, getting him up and helping him dress every morning, until his condition worsened further and he needed to be in a nursing home. She must have mourned, for her husband's sake and her own, the complete loss of his independence and mental health in such a few short years and before Harry was even old enough to retire. The couple never had a chance to share and enjoy their retirement years, a sad reality Harry would no longer be able to grasp but so painful for his grieving wife.

Unlike a major stroke or severe head injury, which inflicts its brain damage all at once, "most illnesses that cause dementia do their damage gradually, so the effects are not seen suddenly," explain Nancy L. Mace and Peter V. Rabins, best-selling authors of *The 36-Hour Day*, an updated and comprehensive reference book on understanding dementia, a book with 416 pages of knowledge and valuable advice for caregivers.

What facts and statistics have to offer is perspective: "Severe memory loss is *never* a normal part of growing older," continue Mace and Rabins. "According to the best studies available, 8 to 10 percent of older people have a severe intellectual impairment, and 10 to 15 percent have milder impairments. The diseases that cause dementia become more prevalent in people who survive into their 80s and 90s, but 50 to 70 percent of those who live to age 90 never experience significant memory loss or other symptoms of dementia."[6]

Most folks who have not yet reached the middle of their eighth decade, when dementia is more likely, will not exhibit severe memory problems. I need to strike another cautionary note, however, and emphasize that even someone relatively young and physically strong can be failing mentally. Like Bella in the story that follows, your loved one may seem to be living independently quite well—until you begin to notice willful and reckless behaviors that raise and wave red flags. This can happen suddenly or, as with the case of Bella, gradually.

BELLA

Bella is a 77-year-old woman whose lifelong devotion to physical fitness continues with daily walks, yoga, and routine participation in spinning and other aerobic exercise classes at her gym. In my opinion, she is an example of a person who may have developed dementia after a lifetime of chronic stress that is known to damage neurons, but whose physical health may have slowed the development and masked the symptoms of her cognitive decline. She has been remarkably resilient despite suffering decades of emotional pain.

Bella's exercise habits may also have delayed the onset of her memory problems and overall cognitive decline. Her healthy eating and fitness activities probably explain why she has been able to live independently even up to the present, when she now demonstrates cognitive loss.

She was only in the tenth grade when her mother had to be hospitalized with schizophrenia. Her dad, working hard to support six children, allowed Bella and her sister to quit school to care for their two youngest siblings, who otherwise would have had to go live with relatives in states far away. She married at 18, had a son, and endured the turmoil and distress of staying with an alcoholic husband until their boy finished high school. Meanwhile, Bella earned her GED, attended community college, and went on to graduate from the University of Maryland.

"Bella's life was always extremely stressful," said her much younger brother, in a recent interview. "Although she moved to Florida to start a new life," Marco explained, "the next man she loved and lived with for more than 30 years [like her first husband] eventually became an alcoholic. Bella constantly worried about and tried to deny or minimize Ben's drinking—even when she'd find hidden beer cans or when he'd go on binges and come home from work in the middle of the day, reeking of alcohol and going to sleep."

In spite of many challenges in her personal life, Bella maintained a daily exercise routine and owned her own business for a time. For many years, she worked capably in positions of high responsibility as an office manager, frugally funded a sizeable personal retirement account, and earned two good pensions.

Bella was 72 when her second husband died. During the following year, Marco and other family members noticed Bella's forgetful episodes but attributed them to the stress of Ben's sad decline from liver disease. She was grieving. Most people in the earlier phases of a mourning process experience a diminished ability to concentrate and at times are so preoccupied with loss that their working memory suffers. Marco knew these things about how people heal and expected that over time his sister's thinking and remembering abilities would gradually return to normal. "But as it got longer and longer after Ben's death," Marco told me, "Bella's memory problems got worse and worse."

In the past five years, in fact, Bella increasingly has shown many cognitive and behavioral changes that *should have* raised red flags and did. "She would schedule appointments, get the time and dates confused, miss the appointments such as for grief counseling—then argue about it and blame the mistake on the clinic staff," Marco explained.

After church, although Bella and her sister's family had long gone to Sunday breakfast at the same place, Bella would forget where they were to meet and how to get there. For Thanksgiving dinner—always at her sister's place or nephew's house, locations with which she was also very familiar—Bella arrived an hour late. She had driven 30 miles in the wrong direction and gotten lost.

"You had to tell Bella two or three times that we are all going to Carrabba's Restaurant on Saturday," Marco recalls. "A few minutes later she would ask, 'Where did you say we're going? Oh, yes, Carrabba's.' Then the day would come to meet for that family dinner and she wouldn't be there. Someone would call her and she hadn't remembered it at all."

Most upsetting to her brother and others aware of the problem was Bella's poor judgment in meeting and sharing personal information with men she met through online dating sites. "One guy who lived 20 miles away, at their first meeting was invited to come stay overnight at her house," remembers Marco. "Bella naively said that she meant it 'just for convenience, not for sex.'

Fortunately, he was a decent man who picked up on her vulnerability and declined."

"You don't know me," said the stranger to Bella. "You shouldn't invite guys back."

Bella was not so lucky when a man she met online told her a sad story about a sick child and talked her into sending him a check for $500. In one of the siblings' frequent long-distance phone conversations, Bella told Marco about the "great e-mail exchanges" she was having with this stranger who said he was from overseas. He also wrote flattering things about how fit and trim Bella looked in her posted photos, said he wanted to meet her, and Bella sent him another check to pay for his air travel. When she went to the airport to meet him, the man never showed up.

Both checks were cashed in Philadelphia, not in an overseas location. Having her bank account number, this man began to deposit money into Bella's account and was trying to withdraw larger amounts. Many banking problems resulted that took months to resolve, requiring help from the FBI, bank officials, and the police.

At breakfast one Sunday with her family, Bella casually disclosed that she was planning to fly to a city 300 miles away to spend the weekend with still another man she met while surfing online dating sites. "Bella seemed oblivious to any of the risks involved," Marco recalled. "When we tried to talk her out of it, she got very defensive and told us that she was an adult and this was none of our business. We said, 'We know that but please let us know where you'll be staying, his name and phone number.'"

Bella was irritated and resistant. "We just want to know where you will be," Marco pleaded, "so at least if something happens, we'll be able to come and help you."

Finally, Bella's loving nephew, Rick, got involved and talked his aunt out of the needed information. After her plane took off for the weekend rendezvous she was determined to have, Rick called this latest stranger, as did Marco shortly thereafter. "We wanted to show that her family was concerned," Marco explained, "so this guy would know that we weren't going to allow her to be isolated."

The man seemed gracious in response to Marco and his nephew's phone calls. If he thought their calls were odd or more than a bit puzzling, he didn't let on. "I'm a nice man," said the fellow on the phone, whose house was where Bella would soon be staying from Thursday to Sunday. "I'm divorced. I have two adult children. I'm from Israel. I have a business in Miami. Bella and I have been talking in e-mails and on the phone for a few months."

Speaking as if to offer more reassurance, "I know who you are," the man in Miami told Marco. "Bella has told me about you and your whole family."

And as they continued to talk, Marco realized that "Bella had casually revealed—to this man she hardly knew—the names of our family members, where everyone lived and worked, and the names of our children."

As it turned out, Bella was very lucky a second time in that she was dealing with an honorable man. She came back from Miami complaining that he mostly went to work every day and left her alone and feeling bored in his apartment.

After this latest incident about a year ago, Marco's level of exasperation reached its peak. Living in another state, a thousand miles away, made him increasingly weary and upset. He phoned Bella and asked her to promise that she would quit the dating sites. "Bella," Marco said, his heart pounding, "you shouldn't be telling all this personal information to people you don't even know! You told him our kids' names? And the last guy got all your bank information! What you are doing is *dangerous*! There are people waiting to take advantage of you, who literally go to websites to find older, vulnerable people to take advantage of, in any way they can. I get too worried and stressed out about you! I can't keep calling if you won't stop talking to and meeting these strange men."

Finally, Bella said, "I'm not going to do this anymore."

Understandably, Marco still worries. While relieved that she is probably no longer on the dating websites, he doesn't know for sure. He recognizes that Bella isn't the person she used to be. She was bright, respected, and capable at her workplace, and at home a published photographer and an artist who did many lovely paintings and drawings of nature scenes. "Now," Marco says, somberly, "Bella is often agitated and anxious, sometimes paranoid, and more and more argues with and isolates herself from family members."

Everyone is always together when Marco's family travels to Florida several times a year. Recently, when they all visited, Bella asked him who that good-looking guy was who (in her mind) seemed to be attracted to her. It hurt Marco a lot to have to say, "Bella, that's my son! It's your nephew, Marco Junior."

For all the family, the problem is that Bella's cognitive impairments now severely cloud her thinking and judgment. She sees herself as doing "just fine" on her own and reacts with anger when anyone suggests otherwise.

Marco admires Bella for her resilience, strength, many talents, and accomplishments in life. Losing their mother to mental illness was hard for all of them, so Marco and his siblings have had to become resilient, too. Still, he sees the particular hardships that Bella had to overcome to complete her education, become successful in her work, develop her artistic talents, and cope with five decades of loving two good men whose lives were eventually lost to alcoholism. Marco respects and doesn't judge Bella, but he wishes she could have been happier, loves her, and cherishes the many good times they've shared. He will always be grateful for the sacrifices Bella and Elena made and the caregiving they gave him and their siblings as children when the older girls were still so young themselves.

THE IMPORTANCE OF PLANNING AHEAD
BEFORE IT'S TOO LATE

It's hard for Marco and his wife to live a thousand miles away, unable to do much more than talk by phone. Because Bella's progressive dementia causes her at times to be so difficult and argumentative, there was a period of time when they didn't talk at all. These days Marco tries to call Bella regularly, whenever he can reach her. He tries as best he can to stay calm, to speak with kindness, and answer the same questions over and over again.

Recently Bella called her sister Elena to say, "I just found $5,400 in my checking account and I don't know where it came from." As it turned out, Bella had paid a tax bill, and the check bounced for insufficient funds, so she transferred money from a savings into a checking account—but she didn't remember why it was there. Not long ago, Bella called Elena again, "I'm really upset! I was supposed to meet you at St. Edwards today!"

"Bella," Elena replied. "I've been sick for four months! I haven't been *able* to go to church."

Increasingly, Marco is realizing that *red flags are everywhere*: "She is incapable of learning new things with her cell phone, so lately she turns it off and it's very difficult for us to get in touch with her. We rarely get responses anymore to our messages sent in texts, e-mails, or left on her answering machine."

Bella has been able to live independently, although not for much longer. What has made it possible to continue to live on her own this long is the structured life she leads. Bella begins the day with a walk on the beach, showers, eats breakfast, goes to the gym for 90 minutes, showers again, and eats another healthy meal. "As long as she does not deviate from these routines," her brother explains, "Bella's life is still rewarding.

"I feel sad for her," Marco says, nearing the end of our conversation. "Until now, I've mostly been okay with where she is. I'm pleased that Bella still has a life. She has things she enjoys. But I'm worried that she will put herself in danger. She is vulnerable to people who would take advantage of her. I worry about her getting lost."

Marco knows that "if we lose my sister Elena to the cancer she's battling, someone else in Florida (probably Elena's son, Rick) will need to step up to look out for Bella's safety and well-being." Marco talks often now with Bella's son, Aaron. They share the mutual frustration of living in Baltimore, too far away to become caregivers themselves.

It was Aaron's idea that Rick should have a key to Bella's house, until such time as Aaron and others in the family can persuade Bella to move into an as-sisted living facility or get paid help at home. They hope to build on the fact that Bella once mentioned a nearby assisted living facility, thinking that if they present it as Bella's own idea, she may be more open to making the move.

Being mentally, socially, and physically active for many years gave Bella the strength and good health needed to face extraordinary challenges and cope with a chronically stress-filled life. That she is still physically active at 77 is how she stays fit, finds pleasure in nature's beauty, and experiences enjoyment from the exercise that lifts her spirits. Living a structured life also has helped her cope. Regardless of her worsening memory and behavioral problems, per-haps in terms of her *physical* health Bella is a role model for finding the best life within reach—under increasingly difficult circumstances.

Unfortunately, Bella is not a role model for planning ahead for a fate that may befall any of us if and when we become no longer able to keep ourselves safe and our financial resources protected. Each of us needs to establish while still sufficiently healthy and young several important legal documents this book will discuss in a later chapter: a personal and durable power of attorney, advance medical directive, last will and testament, and a living revocable trust.

Long before becoming impaired or vulnerable in our own elder years, we need to be having matter-of-fact, frank conversations with our spouse, adult children, siblings, or others on whom we will rely in the event of physical or cognitive disability. We need to be thinking ahead and realistically discussing various options concerning where we could live, if we need to move to assisted living, or how it might be possible to age in place with family assistance or paid nursing support. We should be saving wisely for retirement, which is why it is not a good idea to take out a second mortgage or cosign for a child or a grandchild's college education. It is also smart to consider getting long-term care insurance during our 50s (after that it becomes increasingly expensive), further helping to protect our loved ones from becoming financially burdened by our elder care.

Bella's story is a powerful reminder, too, of how many red flags are missed by well-meaning loved ones. Family members often either can't or won't see the warning signs of dementia—possibly because they fear the conflict they'll have to deal with to convince their loved one to get help *and* the responsibility they'll have to carry once those warning signs are acknowledged.

SOME ADDITIONAL RED FLAGS

Some of the signs and symptoms below, associated with impairments in daily living and brain function, may be present and others not at all. *These behaviors also may be present some days and not on others, indicating "that damaged nerve cells, like a loose light bulb, connect sometimes and fail other times."*[7]

"It's . . . not necessarily forgetting where your keys are. It's forgetting what keys are for."[8] Putting things in odd places, like cookies in the underwear drawer or eyeglasses in the refrigerator. Misplacing things, then accusing someone of stealing and other paranoid or far-fetched ideas. Here are some of the red flags I have noticed and others working in and writing about elder care have noted:

- Completely forgetting a long conversation had just yesterday, as if all these topics had never been discussed, uncharacteristically forgetting an adult child's birthdate, or not being able to follow the rules of a familiar game[9]
- Getting lost when driving to a familiar place, disoriented as to where the kitchen pantry is, or confused about how to exit a grocery store
- Losing interest in activities once meaningful or greatly enjoyed and avoiding people for fear of embarrassing oneself
- Being unable to do tasks which once came easily and were done well, like doing the laundry, balancing a checkbook, making coffee, preparing and following a grocery list, or signing birthday cards to grandchildren

- Saying things that don't make sense or that seem puzzlingly mean, inappropriate, or odd
- Wandering or showing apathy, a significant depression, frequent irritability, or combativeness
- Engaging in socially inappropriate, disinhibited behaviors, hyperorality (putting many or odd things in one's mouth), or compulsive, ritualistic behaviors
- Becoming gradually more impaired in daily functions that involve memory, self-care tasks, and putting words together coherently, or withdrawing from interactions with family and friends
- Not just forgetting but forgetting repeatedly and forgetting what previously would have been unforgettable: losing track of the day, month, season, or year, one's state or town, or being unable to name the current president of the United States
- Having trouble accurately judging the amount of space in between persons or objects or walking with a greatly slowed pace and shortened stride
- Having significant difficulty with object naming, word comprehension, word finding, or grammar

OPTIMAL AGING

Who wants to be just normal? In the words of physician Christiane Northrup, "I want to be *optimal*—not normal!" In her 2015 television program on PBS, *Glorious Women Never Age*, she gives good advice: "Instead of being fearful and instead of feeling anxious, reject the notion that age changes your value!"[10]

In the next chapter, I will discuss ways to combat the unconscious ageist beliefs that can become a self-fulfilling prophecy leading to feeling and acting much older than our chronological years. This will explain why I hope my students, friends, and adult daughters will never hear me say, "I'm having a senior moment," or make an excuse for myself by saying, "I guess I'm just getting old." I will not attribute an ache or pain to my age instead of honestly acknowledging the need to increase the physical activity level in my life to stay limber and fit. I may ask a fellow traveler whether he'll please put my heavy luggage in the overhead storage bin on the airplane, but—without acting helpless—I will just say thanks. People of all ages have neck or back issues, athletic injuries, or occasional memory lapses such as forgetting a name, as was mentioned earlier. And anyone over 40 can feel a little stiff when getting up after spending hours at a time sitting at a computer or watching TV.

It is so important not to yield our lives over to our Western culture's stereotypical ideas about growing older. From research findings we know that people often become in their senior years the persons they envisioned themselves becoming when 20 or more years younger, in their 30s, 40s, and 50s.[11] While it is more difficult in later adult life to reject ageist stereotypes, it's never too late to make a conscious decision to quit using "getting older" as an explanation for behaving a certain way or as an excuse. It's not that we can't ask for and graciously accept help from others when it is needed; we just don't have to attribute so many situations and personal experiences to whatever age we happen to be.

YOU CAN BE REALISTIC *AND* OPTIMISTIC

We can adopt the attitude of having much of value to contribute to our loved ones and community. As of this writing, the average age of the current justices of the US Supreme Court is 69. Astronaut and senator John Glenn was 77 when he traveled for the last time into space for NASA. Lillian Carter was 68 when she served in the Peace Corps in India; her son, former president Jimmy Carter, and his wife, Rosalynn, at 91 and 88, are still active (through the nonprofit Carter Center) in working to stop the spread of parasitic disease in 11 countries across Africa and the Americas. In July 2016, 92-year-old former First Lady Barbara Bush was recognized for 35 years of promoting literacy projects, on the occasion of the twenty-fifth anniversary of the National Literacy Act, for which former president George H. W. Bush credited his wife.

Pope Francis still travels worldwide, at the age of 79, challenging hundreds of thousands of people in every country along the way to work to combat poverty, address the causes of climate change, and create a more just world. Vice President Joe Biden, at the age of 73, led a national effort in the fight against cancer that continues beyond the 2016 election. Bernie Sanders garnered millions of votes, at age 74, running for the presidency of the United States of America. Beatles star Paul McCartney, writes Chris Kelly in the *Washington Post*, has gone from "Fab Four to spry 74," and is still doing concert tours that show off his stamina.[12] Morgan Freeman (79)—who started his movie career at 50—is a costar with Michael Caine (83) and Alan Arkin (82) in the 2017 comedy, *Going in Style*. Still thriving also are singers Joan Baez (75), Tina Turner (76), and Diahann Carroll (80). Movie icon and the author of at least two best-selling memoirs, Sidney Poitier (89), remains active and enjoys playing with his grandchildren and great-grandchildren: Poitier's philosophy is, "If your only goal in life is to improve yourself, then you're doing well."[13] In the next chapter, I'll tell you about a woman I interviewed who is still thriving at 108.

Of course, there *are* things over which we have no control, events that can rob us of our physical health or cognitive abilities, including genetic vulnerabilities that may trigger certain illnesses and other unfortunate medical events that may yet befall us. The odds, however, are still in our favor. It is both appropriate to those odds and the wisest choice to make for the sake of our quality of life for each of us to *choose* to look to the future with optimism. "Your beliefs and expectations about your aging," Dr. Northrup reminds us, "are far more powerful than your genes or environment."[14]

Although I share Dr. Northrup's upbeat approach to getting older, to say that attitudes are "*far* more powerful" may be an overstatement. Our genetic and other biological vulnerabilities sometimes *are* more forcefully determinative than our beliefs. Still, what brings joy and vitality to our lives is living hopefully and taking charge of the ways we think and live as earnestly as possible. I often say to my college students, including many who are of retirement age, "As you expect to experience an experience, so you will experience that experience. Therefore, guard yourself against negative, pessimistic, shortsighted, and self-defeating expectations!"

CHAPTER

4

Aging as Successfully as Possible—Both You and Your Loved One

You can get too old to enjoy life. I never got that old.
—Verona Johnston, age 114, quoted in "Meet the Oldest American,"
by Wendy Cole-Worthington,

Caregiving is so physically tiring and mentally stressful that, at times, you may feel much older than your actual age. You may not be enjoying your life very much these days. Perhaps it's hard to imagine what "successful aging" could mean for you, let alone for your elderly loved one. What helps many people deal with hard times—and may help you—is to look at your life as a story unfolding over many years, with challenges and new opportunities all along the way. Getting the big picture often provides comfort, insight, and hope. We all live our lives in *stages*, with good times and bad, high points and hardships. We probably have more control than we think over how soon we grow old and to what extent we feel well or satisfied with our lives.

THE FOUR AGES OF LIFE

The First Age is childhood and the teen years. The Second Age is the time when we work for a living, raise children, and build strong relationships with family members, friends, and coworkers. During this Second Age, what is called "crystallized intelligence" (vocabulary, logical reasoning, accumulated knowledge, and good judgment gained from experience) grows steadily.[1] The 40s, 50s, and early 60s are often a time of peak performance, creativity, and high achievement in our occupations or community service activities. If you are in this age range, you have many more resources for strength and problem solving than you may realize.

In western Europe and North America, researchers who study human development across the lifespan, including the distinguished psychologist Laura E. Berk, are shattering many widely held beliefs about aging and thus have needed new ways to describe the phase of life previously known as "old age." In recently published textbooks and scientific papers, the Third Age—late adulthood—is often described as "young old age" and the Fourth Age as "old old age."

This Third Age—roughly from ages 65 to 79 or older—is increasingly defined as a period of new goal setting, personal fulfillment, and generativity (a time of giving to others).[2] "At the individual level," explains psychologist Stephen F. Barnes, "the Third Age can last a few years or as much as two decades or more." These are "The Golden Years of Adulthood," he writes, in an article by that title. In these years he calls "golden," while one is still in good physical and psychological health, there are "rich opportunities for self-fulfillment" in activities that give purpose to one's life.[3]

Whether you are in the Second Age (younger than 65) or Third Age, providing respectful, kind, supportive caregiving to your impaired elderly loved one can be a deeply rewarding experience that adds special meaning to your life—especially if you remain mindful of your own needs for self-care and support.

Wellesley College professor Paul Wink, who has studied happiness across the decades of people's lives asks, "Is the Third Age the Crown of Life?"[4] In my own research, I've found countless resilient people in every life stage, including children growing up in extreme poverty or victimized by abuse. Age 50 and beyond, however, may be the *best* time of life for those who have faced and overcome harsh life experiences, have remained as active as possible despite coping with illnesses or loss, are compassionate toward others and insightful when reflecting on their own motives and behavior. Life after 60 is also good when age brings wisdom, a personal sense of well-being, and life satisfaction. Welcome news is the fact that our intelligence as measured by IQ stays pretty much the same from age 20 all the way to age 75, and thankfully our accumulated knowledge goes with us into late life and often into old old age.

Then comes the Fourth Age—old old age—typically the time of diminished physical strength and needing care.[5] People without dementia can still learn new things, but much more slowly over time, with considerable repetition and patience required. This period generally starts sometime during the 80s, although the Fourth Age may begin before age 60 because of a rarer (early-onset) form of Alzheimer's, multiple strokes, substance abuse, or severe head injuries.

Life often becomes increasingly stressful for the 80 percent of persons from ages 85 to 100 or more who suffer losses in three or more areas that include "vision, hearing, strength, functional capacity, illness, and cognition," write Jacqui Smith and Paul Baltes, two of the esteemed authors of *The Berlin Aging Study*. "In advanced old age, individuals may be pushed to the limits of their adaptive psychological capacity."[6] Sadly, because of harsh living conditions and inadequate medical care in developing countries and among the poor in developed nations, people often lose their health and suffer a severely diminished ability to cope, long before having a chance to grow old.

A noteworthy fact is that "the prevalence of dementia is about 50 percent in 90-year-olds."[7] Nonetheless, some form of frailty and reliance on others for caregiving is the eventual fate of most people who live into old old age, and too often this frailty results in a severe impairment in the person's quality of life. *What is most needed to counter the frail elderly person's feelings of extreme vulnerability and to maintain the will to live "is the feeling that there is at least one person one can trust and rely on for emotional support in times of need."*[8]

While arthritis, hip fractures, other health problems, and dementia are common (especially Alzheimer's disease after age 85), explain physician researchers Vaillant and Mukamal, such maladies should not be seen as inevitable. "Most mental deterioration before age 80 reflects disease, not the normal aging process [and] . . . increasingly, successful aging is not an oxymoron."[9] Indeed, according to their research, not only is "successful aging" not a combination of contradictory words: It's an increasingly realistic, achievable goal.

Putting into perspective what are one's chances of physical disability or dementia along the lifespan, Vaillant and Mukamal continue, "73 percent of elderly people report no disability between ages 73 to 84 and even after age 85, a remarkable 40 percent remain fully functional." Even more encouraging, report these authors who study successful aging, it is true that "after 30, our ability to recall proper names steadily declines, but . . . [that] does not predict dementia."[10]

Researchers say there is no greater time of variability in physical and mental capability across the lifespan than from young old age to old old age and the end of life, because people thrive in good health or struggle with poor health in so many different ways and at different ages. We grow old sooner or later, more able or more impaired than others because of illnesses partly resulting from inherited genes (diabetes, Alzheimer's, cardiovascular or other diseases) interacting with our socioeconomic status, level of education, race or ethnicity, and the choices we make (excessive alcohol use, smoking, high-fat diets, inactivity), as well as from exposure to chronic stress, infections, environmental toxins, or head injuries.

Life does not provide a level playing field in that some people are much more vulnerable to mental and physical disability than others. It is also true, however, that the choices we make in life often can offset *many* vulnerabilities, increase our longevity, and improve the quality of our lives. Although lots of things happen to us that are beyond our control, we still have choices. In ways that I will continue to discuss throughout this book, our family, friends, religious or moral beliefs, the community support we receive, and even the way we think about our lives and the decisions we make help to determine our fate.

The good news is that even moderate exercise—almost immediately—makes us feel better, buffers our stress, and begins to reduce our stroke risk and improve heart and lung function. Aerobic exercise also contributes greatly to brain health. A study of older adults whose healthy brains were scanned at age 69 and scanned again at age 78 showed that walking six to nine miles each week *increased* the walkers' gray matter over a nine-year period when an older person's gray matter would be expected to decrease. In fact, those in the control group who were not habitual walkers during the study *did* lose gray matter and developed dementia at twice the rate of the walkers who averaged 30 minutes daily.[11]

WHEN OLD AGE IS IN THE EYE OF THE BEHOLDER

Young adults (18 to 29) surveyed by the Pew Research Center believe that most people become old at age 60, while middle-aged adults set the mark at 70. People who themselves are 65 or older, however, think becoming old doesn't happen until age 74. More than one-third of 65 to 74 year olds say they *feel* younger than their actual age by 10 to 20 years.[12]

Researchers have also found that older adults who feel younger and think of themselves as younger than their chronological age are happier, more satisfied with life, and are more likely to engage in healthy eating, exercise, and stimulating activities. Of course, it works both ways: healthy behaviors lead to better physical functioning and a greater sense of personal control over one's fate.[13]

False generalizations and many distorted assumptions about aging include the idea that growing old equates to illness, loneliness, depression, an end to sexual activity, and an inability to drive. In reality, according to the Pew study, only "about one in five [adults ages 65 and older] say they have a serious illness, are not sexually active, or often feel sad or depressed. About one in six report they are lonely or have trouble paying bills. One in seven cannot drive." And, although any number in this category is too high, fewer than most people think (one in ten) say they feel they "aren't needed" or are a "burden to others." All of these atypical problems (except for sexual inactivity) are challenges more often faced by older adults with low incomes.[14] When well enough to share physical intimacy with an available and consenting partner or comfortable with the idea of pleasuring themselves, a majority of adults ages 65 to 85 are sexually active at least two or three times per month.[15] For this reason, I often remind family members and paid caregivers, whether at home or in nursing facilities, to respect and protect the privacy of young old and old old adults, and not to judge them if they masturbate or discount their need for shared romantic affection or sexual intimacy.

While young and middle-aged adults *expect* memory loss to be a problem they will have to deal with at age 65 and beyond, only about 25 percent of adults 65 and older say they are *experiencing* some form of memory loss. In fact, an optimistic, count-my-blessings approach to life by far is more common than negativity. About 70 percent of older adults answer positively when asked whether they are "enjoying more time with family," 60 percent report that they "get more respect and feel less stress than when they were younger," and more than half say that they appreciate having "more time to travel and do volunteer work."[16] Studies also show that even among the old old (80s and older), a mere 1 percent "say their lives have turned out worse than they expected."[17]

THE IMPORTANCE OF REJECTING AGEISM

According to researcher Becca Levy's work, reported in *JAMA*, seniors who expect aging to be a positive experience are "44 percent more likely to fully recover from a bout of disability." Yale professor Levy further found that "those with positive age stereotypes lived 7.5 years longer than those with negative stereotypes."[18] Citing these studies in the *New York Times*, Judith Graham explains that "positive age stereotypes are associated with a greater sense of control . . . [as well as an] enhanced seniors' sense of self-efficacy," allowing older adults to "remain captains of their own ship."[19]

We need to "ditch ageist stereotypes," declares retirement policy expert Ros Altmann in a recent article for the *Guardian*. Labels such as "frail, past it, over the hill, and decrepit diminish the value of older adults," she continues. "Ageist terms should be as unacceptable as racist or sexist ones." Such prejudicial attitudes need to be challenged as false, damaging, and "a waste of time for all of us."[20]

Ageist stereotypes negatively impact how older adults view themselves, as seen in a study led by psychologist Dana Kotter-Grühn of North Carolina State University. "Older adults in good health felt older after being exposed to negative stereotypes," and those in bad health felt even worse.[21] It takes a conscious effort not to "buy in" to society's negative age-related stereotypes or presume them appropriate and impose them on ourselves.

When I was in my late 20s, I lived in a row house in Baltimore City next door to a judge and his wife who were probably in their mid-60s. Every time I stopped by their porch to visit, they talked about subjects I swore I would never talk about when I got to be their age. The couple didn't look very old to me; they had no obvious disabilities, but every topic they brought up seemed to relate to physical complaints and their rather intimate bodily functions, "regularity" and that sort of thing! They were the opposite of the much older couple whose row house shared a fire wall with mine: these folks were in their 80s, full of interesting stories, and were generous with acts of kindness directed my way.

Continuing to work full time after becoming a college professor decades ago, I realize that my students will only wonder how "old" I am in any kind of disparaging way if I give them some reason to do so by the attitudes and behaviors I project. "I still love teaching," I tell my students, "after starting out as a 'hippie' and being here for more than 30 years." (Not calling attention to what "more" in actual years means, I don't wear my 45-year lapel pin, which is larger than a quarter and happier left at home.) Because I genuinely *do* love this work and believe with a passion in our educational mission, I dress everyday like a person going in for a job interview, walk into the room with an upbeat attitude, and move about the classroom with energy and excitement. At any age in life, even when physical disabilities become part of our lives, I believe that others will define us not just by what we talk about and how we carry ourselves, but even more so according to how we treat *them*, and whether we follow the Golden Rule.

We become "old" in other people's eyes when we stop enjoying life, no longer live with purpose, turn inward, fill our conversations with complaints, and don't show that we still care about others and *their* well-being. As a teacher, I want my words and actions to demonstrate that what I care about most is my students' success—in my course, their other courses, their personal lives, and future occupations. Many already are parents or grandparents, while others will start their families in just a few years. My goal is to challenge each student to "See what you can be," which is our college motto. For many individuals of all ages, their last door of opportunity may be getting a quality, affordable, community college education. As mentioned earlier, I work hard to learn each student's name as soon as possible. I want to emphasize that each life matters to me.

In her 2014 best-selling book, *Aging Backwards*, and on her fitness show on public television, Miranda Esmonde-White asks and answers a question most people older than 40 are eager to hear, "Do you want to know how to look 10 years younger? Stand up straight!"[22] Like many others who spend too many hours each week sitting in front of a computer, I have a tendency to walk with the slumping shoulders Miranda describes. I try to be mindful of her advice as I pace around the classroom, walk down hallways and around our home, and especially when I start the day walking the family dog. "Standing tall" makes a person *feel* younger, projects strength and self-confidence.

At any age, practicing good posture is beneficial to back and neck health, too, and can lift up our self-esteem. From personal experience, I also know that Esmond-White's "classical stretch" exercises foster agility, improve balance, and strengthen feelings of well-being.

LEARNING FROM THE MASTERS

Displayed in my study for more than 30 years is a large, colorfully framed piece of wall art bearing a quotation in letters two inches tall. There, to remind me of a life lesson I never want to forget, are words spoken by the world-famous cellist Pablo Casals: "The main thing in life is not to be afraid to be human."

Even as an 80-year-old, Casals was not afraid to engage life fully and to continue setting goals for himself. "When a young student asked why he continued to practice so hard," Casals answered, "Why? This is simple. Because I want to get better."[23]

In the medical journal *Gerontology*, the internationally esteemed researcher Paul Baltes and his associate Jacqui Smith relate the Casals story above to illustrate a concept called "self-plasticity," meaning our "substantial latent potential for better [physical and mental] fitness in old age." Baltes and his wife Margret's research additionally demonstrates the good news that—in the Third Age—there are "more and more people who age successfully," experience "high levels of emotional and personal well-being," and use "effective strategies to master the gains and losses of late life."[24]

Another widely acclaimed 80-year-old musician, classical pianist Arthur Rubinstein, offers the Baltes' favorite example of a coping skill essential to successful aging: a life-management skill known as *selective optimization with compensation*. "When Rubinstein was asked how he continued to be such an excellent concert pianist, he named three reasons. He played fewer pieces, but practiced them more often, and he used contrasts in tempo to simulate faster playing than he in the meantime could master." By reducing his repertoire (selection), Rubinstein could practice each piece more (optimization), and make up for the fact that his aging fingers couldn't move as rapidly (compensation).[25]

Describing "the art of life in old age," Paul and Margret Baltes offer a hopeful, powerful lesson for caregivers and care recipients alike: what successful aging is all about is finding "a new, usually smaller territory that is cared for with similar intensity as in the past."

Akin to the lesson to be gained from Rubinstein's life is the wisdom author Bert Brim provides in telling the story of his father, who lived to the age of 103. In his book entitled, *Ambition: How We Manage Success and Failure Throughout Our Lives*, Brim says that as a younger man his dad farmed a large acreage. At 75, lacking the mobility of his younger years, his dad hired someone else to do the farming and shifted his own energies to overseeing a spacious garden. By age 90, when his hearing and sight were failing and his mobility became severely impaired, Brim's dad focused on his houseplants. Some years later, his dad's goal setting and feelings of well-being continued: he cared for the flowers on the window ledge near the chair where he sat most of the day.

How might *you* conserve but maximize *your* energies, select and stay involved in activities that bring *you* pleasure, personal fulfillment, and stress relief? And in what ways does the above story of the farmer also shed light on how your impaired elderly loved one might be helped to continue meaningful activities in smaller, more manageable ways?

DOWNING KAY: BORN IN 1907, STILL AGING WELL

"I got a tip that, while Downing Kay is not a baseball fan, she might be the only person in the Baltimore region who was alive when the Chicago Cubs last won the World Series," wrote Dan Rodricks, in the *Baltimore Sun*. "Almost 109 and Still Going Strong, Honey," was Rodrick's headline. He interviewed her just days before the Cubs' dramatic win in game 7.[26]

She was 100 years old when her son died and 108 when I interviewed her. Her daughter, age 70, had visited from Florida the previous week. "It's probably not a good idea at my age to get new hearing aids," she chuckled, "but when my daughter was here, we got new hearing aids."

Downing Kay has fond memories of courtship, marriage, and parenting, working for several years as a door-to-door polltaker for Gallup, getting her teaching certificate from the normal school (a two-year college), and "loving children" during 20 years as a kindergarten teacher. Mrs. Kay's husband of 46 years, George, passed away several decades ago, after which time she "moved to a condo" and took "church-sponsored group trips with a woman friend to South America, the Black Sea, and England a couple of times."

Since 1995, Downing Kay has made her home in an independent living apartment in the Pickersgill Retirement Community, a nonprofit multilevel care facility in Baltimore. One of her granddaughters, a woman in her mid-50s, comes weekly to pay the bills and do her laundry. A staff member cleans her apartment once a week. Her daughter always stays for a week when she visits four times a year but calls to talk with her every night at seven o'clock. Mrs. Kay is very fond of her daughter-in-law who lives near Washington, DC, close enough to visit fairly often.

Her one-bedroom apartment is an attractive place—decorated with knick-knacks, framed wall art, a coffee table, a couple of sturdy wooden armchairs, and a small couch with pillows and other accessories in various shades of pink. When I arrive to interview her, Mrs. Kay is nicely dressed, like a lady expecting company or ready to go out. She leaves her walker and cane in the entryway and moves about the apartment by steadying herself from one piece of furniture to another. She leads me to a card table and two chairs, knowing I'm there to ask, "What are the keys to aging well?"

Mrs. Kay starts the conversation by describing the dining room where the residents have their evening meals. There she prearranges to have dinner with a different friend every weeknight. Tonight, she tells me, she's having dinner with "a retired nun who always plays poker with the men." She explains that "conversation is a lost art," so she thinks ahead to have interesting topics for discussion and preempt any unseemly table talk. "You don't age well if you talk about your aches and pains," says Mrs. Kay, "and you have to be rather good at keeping your mouth shut. If you're asking questions, you're jerking from others what they don't want to say. Whatever other people are interested in— even if it's a sick dog, be interested in the dog!"

Covering the refrigerator door in the small but cozy apartment's kitchen are photos of her grandchildren, great- and great-great-grandchildren. She tries but is unable to name every one of them for me, on the spot, right then and there; but she stays frequently in touch with these much-loved grandchildren, mostly by phone. Her memory has failed in some ways but is largely intact. Mrs. Kay tells me she enjoyed playing bridge with friends as long as her eyesight lasted and stayed close to her siblings while they were alive, three brothers who died in their 90s and a younger sister who lived to be 100. Using a magnifying glass, Downing Kay still plays Scrabble with another resident of the Pickersgill senior living community who comes to her apartment most Friday nights.

"GROWING AND LEARNING ALL THE TIME"

Mrs. Kay uses a walker to move down the long hallway to activities beyond her own door, including—she explains—the musical programs and speakers who come regularly and the monthly social where "I take wine." She especially looks forward to that one communal daily meal, "where you're dying to talk about what's going on," sharing conversations that "keep me growing and learning all the time."

Noticing that she is remarkably up to date on recent newsworthy events, I ask Mrs. Kay how she manages to be so aware, with macular degeneration having rendered her legally blind for most of the last 20 years. "I don't do much TV," she says, "but I watch the news and I listen to Diane Rehm on NPR." She uses a bright light and magnifying glass to read some things in large print.

Recently, a letter came from her church asking all members to complete an anonymous survey as to whether they approved or disapproved of their minister performing same-sex marriages in the sanctuary. "I thought long and hard about it," she told me, "and I decided, 'Yes.' But I also wrote that I think the gay couples should stay and come to our services—and not just use the church as a place to get married." That someone who was born in 1907 could stretch her mind to embrace the idea of marriage equality in 2015, at the church she still attends, struck me as pretty remarkable.

From her apartment, Downing Kay prays individually as a member of a prayer group, praying by name for people in the church and community who are grieving, ill, or troubled. "I feel close to my Lord," she says. "I'm in prayer a good deal."

One of her favorite friends is "84 but you'd think she's 35, still living in a big house on her own." Another occasional companion is a "92-year-old friend who still drives and will drive me to church, but I need someone to walk with who has a strong arm," she explains.

"*I* have a strong arm," I tell her, and offer to take her to church. I am close in age to her daughter and still work full time, but I am old enough to collect Social Security. "Oh, to be so young as you are!" she exclaims.

By living so long, Mrs. Kay has lost the majority of the people she has loved in her life—including her parents, four siblings, husband, son, and a great many friends. It is only because she reaches out to, shows interest in, and stays close with her younger family members and friends that these strong social connections abide and thrive. She also has made new friends—even after entering her second century of life!

Being able to adapt to changing circumstances is one of the hallmarks of resiliency and successful transitions at every stage along the lifespan. No doubt Mrs. Kay has many age-related physical disabilities, in addition to some memory problems and other limitations. Nevertheless, other than just mentioning in passing that she is nearly blind and virtually deaf without her hearing aids, she did not speak of any of her frailties in our time together. Mrs. Kay is someone who adapts to the things she cannot change and has probably been a person who, at every stage of her life, refuses to feel sorry for herself.

With a palpable sense of humor indicative of accepting the many frustrations and challenges of reaching such an old age, she tells of an elderly man who recently gave a long and eloquent speech at her multilevel care facility, on the subject of the old Wild West. After his speech, this greatly admired historian, like many with age-related memory problems, was disoriented and exasperated when he couldn't remember where he'd parked. "I don't have that problem," said Mrs. Kay with a wry smile. "I don't have a car!"

Extraordinary longevity, studies confirm, runs in families "genetically blessed," especially the 20 percent of US centenarians who smoked and had imperfect eating habits. Most Americans who have lived this long, however, "used their bodies as they were designed and programmed over the millennia: for walking, for working, for being fed from the earth's natural bounty. It makes one wonder whether the next generation of oldsters will last quite as long," write the authors of the *Time* magazine article on people who've lived to be 100. "They will need not just the luck of the genetic draw but also the strength to renounce the lure of fast-food days and couch-potato nights that add yards of lard and shorten life-spans by years."[27]

Of course Mrs. Kay's quality of life and longevity are significantly attributable to having good genes; after all, her parents and all four siblings lived to age 89 or older. In science, it is well established that genes influence hardiness and our risk factors for cancer, heart disease, strokes, and many other diseases including Alzheimer's. Most of us simply don't have that perfect combination of fortunate genes, healthy lifestyle, a strong social support system, access to good medical care when needed, and a plentiful supply of good luck. Regardless, at whatever age we presently are, there are valuable lessons to be drawn from the decades of wise choices and resilient attitudes of this interesting and delightful 108-year-old woman.

What an amazing role model is this person with the unusual but sweet-sounding name of Downing Kay. She is interested in other people but not nosy, careful not to talk only about her own life but does share what is meaningful from her past, and fully engages current topics of interest. She also refuses to focus on the aches and pains associated with aging. Mrs. Kay stays in close contact with her much-cherished family members and friends; she draws strength from her faith, rich supply of fond memories, and new opportunities for learning. She lives with a grateful heart. She is the kind of person that younger people want to spend time with and learn from, in the hope of similarly—at whatever age—growing old with wisdom and grace.

YOU CAN REDUCE YOUR RISK FACTORS FOR DEMENTIA

Even if you are already "getting older," you can improve your chances of aging well. If you smoke, you are doubling your risk of dementia resulting from vascular disease (hypertension, aortic stiffening, a major stroke, or multiple small strokes), and you may be doubling your risk of Alzheimer's disease as well.

Avoid second-hand smoke, too. If you stop smoking, your overall health may begin to improve almost right away.

Alcohol and drugs can have a toxic impact on brain health. As women, our average recommended drink limit is said to be one a day, and for men two drinks daily. Some studies strongly recommend having no more than a couple of drinks a week and no alcohol at all when certain medications have been prescribed. Risk factors for neurocognitive disorders induced by substance use or medications include "older age, longer use, and persistent use past age 50 years."[28]

Diabetes is a vascular risk factor shown in studies to nearly double the risk of dementia, especially among those who suffer from a more severe or longer history of diabetes.[29] Most people with a family history of diabetes or fasting blood sugar level in the danger zone can avoid this chronic illness or successfully control it through diet and exercise with or without medication. Follow your doctor's orders for preventing its onset or treating the diabetes if you already have it, and for treating high blood pressure and high cholesterol.

Physical inactivity is another major risk factor for Alzheimer's disease and vascular dementia. Inactivity both shortens and diminishes the quality of countless lives by significantly contributing to Americans' high rates of obesity, heart disease, diabetes, depression, and cancer. Both animal and human studies demonstrate that regular exercise improves learning, memory, and overall health, and increases brain plasticity and volume. Aerobic exercise, good nutrition, and maintaining a healthy weight will keep us younger than our actual years and especially benefit those who suffer from arthritis, keeping them mobile longer and less likely to become wheelchair bound.

Just as exercise improves the quality and length of our lives, a physically active lifestyle, as we saw in Bella's story, can be a powerful weapon for combating chronic stress, may delay the onset of dementia in a vulnerable person, and can enable a person to remain independent longer than might otherwise be possible. Remember, however, that one need not be the extraordinarily fit person that Bella is or have practiced an active lifestyle for decades. Swimming, gardening, dancing, stretching exercises, yoga, and playing golf or tennis are beneficial at almost any age. In the study cited earlier, showing the impact of regular exercise on older people with healthy brains, the dementia rate was reduced by half—even when the 30-minute daily walk became a routine during the nine years from ages 69 to 78.[30] Scientists at the University of Kansas Alzheimer's Disease Center, in a new study, found that even a "lower dose" of exercise is beneficial. While the more you exercise, the more your endurance and fitness will increase, starting a brisk walking program for just 75 minutes weekly (even after age 65) was shown to improve thinking skills.[31]

If you don't have a dog, maybe you should consider getting one. You'll have an adoring companion to elevate your mood, lift the spirits of the loved one in your care, *and* you'll be forced out of the house several times a day to walk your four-footed friend. I purposely don't have a fenced yard so that I am required to walk our border collie, Panda, in every season and regardless of the weather. Taking a healthy walk first thing in the morning has been proven to be the exercise habit easiest to maintain, and it works for me.

What is the physical activity that will do the most good for *your* overall health? On this, all physicians agree: the best exercise is the exercise that you will keep doing!

CAREGIVER SELF-CARE

As a caregiver, often taxed to the maximum of your mental and physical capabilities, you need recreation and stimulation not only to keep your spirits up in difficult circumstances but also to keep your own brain working well. Researchers have examined many specific leisure activities potentially beneficial in reducing one's risk factors for dementia: learning new and complex things from computer and smart phone applications, studying a foreign language, taking dancing lessons, playing a musical instrument, playing board games or cards, reading or working crossword puzzles, and volunteering in community service activities. While the jury is still out on which particular activities are effective ways to strengthen your brain health, the more activities (in addition to walking) that you do weekly, the better are your chances of remaining mentally sharp.[32] One thing we know with certainty is that such activities provide relief from the stressful work of caregiving, will enrich your life, and can even improve your self-esteem.[33]

THE IMPORTANCE OF SLEEP AND SOCIAL ACTIVITIES

As a caregiver, you need to know that not getting enough sleep has been associated with depression, obesity, a significantly reduced quality of everyday mental functioning, and a gradual cognitive decline over time. Most people need seven to eight hours of quality sleep most nights of the week. Best-selling author and brain expert Dr. Daniel Amen, in *Use Your Brain to Change Your Age*, gives good advice: "Try a warm bath before bed, no television an hour before bed, [or] a sleep-inducing hypnosis CD . . . [A breathing disorder like] sleep apnea doubles a person's risk for Alzheimer's disease, so get a sleep study done if you suspect this could be an issue."[34]

As necessary to maintaining one's mental and physical health as it is to stop smoking, decades of research published in medical journals report that it is *equally important* to stay socially connected. Social isolation is a chronic stressor shown in animal and human studies to lead to a host of bad health outcomes, including accelerating cognitive decline with age.[35]

Interactions of various kinds and conversations with other people beneficially stimulate and require a high level of function in multiple regions of the human brain. Your friends, neighbors, those with whom you worship or engage in social activities, and others who aid you in caregiving or offer companionship—each and all of these persons can foster brain health as well as add meaning and joy to your life.

You may need to ask a family member or hire someone to be a regular caregiver in your place a few hours every day or several afternoons or evenings each week so that you can routinely engage in physical exercise as well as mentally stimulating and socially supportive activities. Think of these activities as stress buffers that provide your brain with nourishment and benefit your overall health.

YOU CAN IMPROVE YOUR LOVED ONE'S QUALITY OF LIFE

Please remember that the person in your care, if able, will be greatly helped by participating in any of the above-mentioned physical, mental, and social activities. Taking your loved one for walks, to the local Y or your gym for a low-impact exercise class in a warm-water pool (often attended by seniors and people recovering from surgery), riding along in the car on errands or for a restaurant meal, attending religious services or concerts and other community events, or participating regularly in "memory care" programs at a local nursing facility—any such stimulating activities and others can be very beneficial. A trip to the hairdresser or barber, a pedicure at home or at a spa, a "picnic" in a lawn chair with a sandwich while sitting anywhere with an open window, on one's own balcony, or at nearby park—all such activities can be of comfort and relieve the monotony of the days.

Almost any form of leisure that involves movement will diminish stiffness, improve mobility, and feel invigorating. When my elderly parents were virtually homebound, either a nursing aide who came several days a week or my sister led them in a variety of stretching exercises they could do from their chairs, then repeatedly walked them around in wide circles through the living room and kitchen. My folks enjoyed the attention and often laughed as my dad marched like a soldier on the arm of the aide or joked with my mother. They both seemed to be having fun.

My mother, throughout her life and until just weeks before her death, loved more than anything to go out for a drive and an ice cream cone. When visiting my folks in Oklahoma and later in Texas, I loved sharing Mama's sheer happiness over simple things and tried always to take her to her favorite ice cream parlor. My own daughters will tell anyone that I am similarly crazy about ice cream in general and ridiculously joyful when stopping at Dairy Queens when we travel. Maybe it's a way of feeling close to my mother, now that she is gone.

While Mama was a person who liked to sit in a car and "watch people," my dad would sit for hours at a time on their tiny porch, smoking cigars and listening to music on his ancient Walkman, punching buttons he could still operate from memory. So when visiting my parents, most of the time I spent with Daddy involved joining him in smoking cigars or working in the yard doing jobs that he "supervised" despite being nearly blind.

After he became a widower, we found him a place to live where the caretakers knew this 95-year-old man needed the music in his room to be playing almost constantly, and where they would watch over him with eagle eyes whenever Daddy wanted to smoke one of his cigars.

If your loved one is in a nursing home or assisted living facility, visiting often and at unexpected times will enable you to observe your elderly spouse, parent, or other family member's living situation and caregivers. When staff members know that someone in the family is faithfully overseeing a loved one's care, they almost inevitably provide better and more attentive care. To the best of his or her ability to walk unassisted, with a cane or walker, staying mobile is essential. In facilities understaffed, with employees insufficiently trained and poorly paid, "care" often amounts to keeping the patients or residents in wheelchairs for hours at a time. Stimulating activities need to be plentifully available, and the residents encouraged and helped to participate in them.

Notice if the television is on in your loved one's room almost constantly, set to stations of a caregiver's preference and annoying or distressing to your loved one. Staff members and their supervisors need to know if your loved one *never liked* watching TV and prefers a quiet atmosphere or be told which programs and types of music are your loved one's favorites. I will talk in a later chapter about such facilities and the many things to watch for that may be causing your family member unnecessary anxiety and agitation, possibly indicating caregiver ineptitude, neglect, or abuse.

Offering words of wisdom and immeasurably valuable advice in their book for family caregivers, Nancy Mace and Peter Rabins emphasize finding the best life within reach for persons with Alzheimer's disease or other types of dementia:

> We already know how to change the quality of life for some people who have dementia: we can make changes that help them to function as well as possible, we can reduce their anxiety and fear, and we can make it possible for them to enjoy some things sometimes . . .
>
> . . . Researchers have observed that people who had previously paced, screamed, and struck out became relaxed and had fewer distressing and disrupting behaviors when they participated in enjoyable activities.[36]

THE QUALITY OF *YOUR* LIFE MATTERS, TOO

To age successfully from whatever age you presently are, you need to think of physical, mental, social, and spiritual self-caring activities not as luxuries but as survival and coping essentials. However much you are devoted to providing quality care to your impaired elderly loved one, you do not owe this person your own premature aging. Loyalty does not require living with near-constant fatigue or compromising your own mental and physical health. The activities I have described represent brain-healthy lifestyle choices and are behaviors that will make you stronger and a more effective caregiver.

In the words of Dr. Amen, "Get healthy for yourself, but also do it for your children and great-grandchildren [or others] who want you around, lucid and vibrant and smiling, to enjoy life with them as long as humanly possible."[37]

Anger, Guilt, and Resentment

Accept the pain, cherish the joys, resolve the regrets; then can come the best benedictions—"If I had my life to live over, I'd do it all the same."
—Joan McIntosh, American writer, born 1943

Feelings of anger and resentment are an almost inevitable response when someone we love is made to suffer from an awful disease like Alzheimer's or because of another person's actions. Whether harm is inflicted accidentally or intentionally, directly or indirectly, strong emotions arise within us that often take months or years to resolve. When bad things happen to good people, as Rabbi Harold Kushner describes in his book by that title, a person of faith often struggles with feelings of anger toward God. Whether we have a secular or spiritual view of the world, senseless suffering leaves many of us clenching and raising a furious fist in the air. How can we not at certain times feel compelled to protest this mysteriously random universe or divinely created world where pain and sorrow are borne by literally billions of innocent human beings?

JOHN'S STORY

Sweet Memories and Difficult Years

John R. says he is "angry at God for making Dorothy sick five years ago. Not that she died. Everybody has to die." He doesn't understand why someone who "was not a criminal or bad person," a person as lovely and loving as his wife of 65 years, "had to get something like that [dementia]." The gradual devastation of the person most precious to him, the ravages wrought by Alzheimer's disease, have shaken but not broken this sturdy 86-year-old family man.

John's anger is understandable, but what he does not resent are the years of tender caregiving he provided for Dorothy. She was the love of his life, the woman he met when he was only 18 and married one year later. He accepts the pain he experienced as her health failed, cherishes the joys they shared for so many years, and considers it a "blessing" that he was able to be her primary caregiver to the end. "At the Cahill Rec Center, there was always live music on Saturday night," he vividly remembers. "We danced a lot [the night they met], and at the last dance I said, 'Can I go home with you on the streetcar?' On East North Avenue then, I walked Dorothy up to her door and gave her a kiss. From then on I was hooked."

After they married, "she got pregnant right away," and their four children were born within 10 years. "I took every test I could to become a building inspector," John recalled. "She was a great mother, always had a nice big supper of roast beef, carrots, and potatoes or pork chops, or chicken livers, and fried onions. We sent the kids through 12 years of Catholic school, bought a Christmas tree farm, and built a house there. We took the three youngest kids, piled into a Ford station wagon, went to Ocean City often, to New York, and out west to the Grand Canyon and Yellowstone."

After the children were grown, his building inspection and senior management positions enabled John to have lunch almost daily with Dorothy. She took one college psychology course after another for personal enrichment and enjoyed telling him what she was learning, sitting alongside students younger than their children. Together they traveled often to faraway conventions for building managers, including to Denver, Miami, Toronto, Washington, and Montreal. Eight grandchildren and five great-grandkids further enriched their lives.

He would need such sweet and happy memories of their life together to sustain him during the increasingly difficult and heartbreaking years of her everworsening illness.

"About seven or eight years ago, when she was driving and I was following behind in my car, it was raining and she pulled over," John sadly recalled. "I got out and went to her on the driver's side."

"I don't know how to turn the windshield wipers on," she said.

"Roll down the window," he answered, "so I can turn them on."

"I don't know how," Dorothy replied.

That incident, and the Sunday at Mass when he saw that she'd forgotten what to do with the Holy Communion wafer, signaled troublesome changes soon to complicate their lives. Not only was her memory failing but her warm, gracious personality was changing, too. Much to John's astonishment, "she was angry, dissatisfied, argumentative with doctors, and even threatened to kill me. I hid the knives and then she'd even forget that she was going to kill me."

John recalled that four years ago, "as she continually got worse, I tried sending Dorothy to an active day care program." Although he is a straight-standing, tall, and fit man who looks to be more in his early 70s than his mid-80s, it was hard for John to get his increasingly frail wife from the wheelchair onto the care facility's bus, the bus would often be late, and the whole situation became unmanageable. He decided to keep her at home.

Dorothy was bedridden the last three years of her life, but John was determined to "get her in the living room every day so she could be in the sunshine." He got a Hoyer Lift, a crane on wheels with a hammock-like sling, that cradled her and enabled John to swing her from the bed into a geriatric wheelchair that reclined. With the Hoyer alone he could turn her over and lay her back down. "I'd feed her and change her diapers and give her snacks. I didn't consider it a chore. It was a blessing to me. Still, it was wearing me down. I tried to hire sitters to help but a lot of the time they didn't show up. There was also a problem with a sitter who stole jewelry from the house and was caught by the bank having altered a $50 check I wrote, making it $1,500."

A Thankful Heart

Gilchrist Hospice, a nonprofit agency in Baltimore that I have worked with professionally on many occasions and know to provide skillful, comprehensive, and compassionate care, came to John's rescue. Dorothy was assessed as having three to six months to live, but "she lasted much longer than that," John told me. After he reached out to them for help, Gilchrist sent a doctor once a month and an LPN who came weekends to bathe and feed Dorothy and provide other personal care.

He will be grateful to his own dying day, John told me, unable to say enough about the support he received. "Gilchrist also came through with respite care: once a month they sent an ambulance to take Dorothy to a nursing home for five days to give me a break, I'd go to Ocean City, and then they'd bring her back. Three months before she died, I had a premonition. I didn't go anymore."

John's sweet memories bring him comfort and help to lift the burden of those long caregiving years, especially when he gets to talk about Dorothy at length with someone who just lets him tell his love story. "We ate out a lot after

I retired or I'd cook. We traveled all over the country." And, holding each other close, over the decades they often danced together around the living room, just as they'd danced together as newly smitten teenagers. "For 55 of the 65 years we were happy," John said, wiping tears away. "In the last years, she forgot who I was and how to kiss, but I'd kiss her anyway."

It was "still a shock" when he "got up at six a.m. on the morning of February 13, 2015, to turn her over" and found that Dorothy had died. "The nurse and a doctor came and the funeral home took her out. I called Johns Hopkins' equipment company and within an hour or two her bed was gone, and the Hoyer crane, and geri chair [geriatric wheelchair]. I gave away her clothes but I'm keeping her love letters and jewelry."

Moving Forward

John is not so mad at God that it keeps him from the church that has given him so much strength and meaning throughout his life. He is also not afraid to try something new and if that doesn't work to try something else. Not long after Dorothy passed away, he "went to the American Legion to a couple of their dances," he told me, but he didn't find the female companionship he was looking for there. "I liked their looks and everything but I just didn't see anyone I was interested in dating."

An inspiration to those who have known him a long time and to me, who only met him recently, John is exhibit A of a recent widower determined to live fully the life that he still has, as long as he can. Always a person who wants to make a contribution to others' lives, since his retirement he has volunteered at a psychiatric hospital, about once a month when Dorothy was alive and weekly since then, where he builds nature trails and benches around the grounds, designs ads for volunteers, does paper work, and whatever else is needed. He swims regularly at the place where his daughter teaches water aerobics. He frequently takes dancing lessons, has lunch twice a week with the same daughter who lives nearby, and enjoys taking regular walks. Three times a week John lifts weights at the League for the Handicapped, where he also visits with and tries to uplift the spirits of people whose difficult life circumstances and significant disabilities remind him that his own life situation is still remarkably good. He is living the best life within reach for him, and thriving at 86.

As often happens with the head of a family who has always been seen by loved ones as "the strong one," it frequently feels to John as if some members of his family have forgotten him. Although he would never tell them so, there are times when he feels resentful. "Sometimes people bring me food, but at night I'm going to be sitting in an empty house. I don't need food. I need company.

"I'm mostly not lonely," John says, referring to how busy he keeps himself during the daytime. Still, he is a man who was accustomed to family life, the first 19 years with his parents, and the next 65 with Dorothy. While he was caring with such devotion for his increasingly forgetful and then frail wife in their last decade together, John's family may have come to think of him as pretty much unavailable or self-sufficient. A man who comes across as fit, active, and much younger than his chronological years, he probably needs to remind the most receptive ones among his adult children and grandchildren that he is *living alone for the first time in his life*. As difficult as it is for John to get beyond feelings of resentment at having to ask for their support, he needs to say to one of his daughters or sons, "I'm doing well in most ways, but the nights are hard. It sure would help if you'd ask your siblings to take turns inviting me to dinner once a week or so." And he can make it a habit to invite one of his adult children or grandchildren to eat out with him, or go to a ball game, or some other event they'd both enjoy.

All I Did Was Listen

During our interview, John shed tears, both happy and sad. He said he'd previously found it hard to cry and seemed to appreciate the opportunity just to be and say whatever he felt. The meeting in my office was about two hours long. As he was leaving, I was touched when John turned to me in the doorway and said, "You've helped me."

"By sharing your story, you've helped me write something that will help a lot of other people," I replied.

A few days later, I woke up in the middle of the night with words in my head. I knew I couldn't go back to sleep until I got the light on, found a pen, and wrote something down. I had to be sure not to forget those words. It was the sentence John had said on his way out.

"In what way did I help him?" I wondered. Interviewing people for my books, I quite deliberately stay in the role of a writer and do not respond as a psychologist or pastoral counselor. I focus on their story. I don't ask probing questions or try to offer comfort or give advice. I simply ask each person to share their caregiving experience, I listen, and I take a lot of notes.

All I did was listen. "You've helped me," he said. John showed me pictures of his wife as a young, then middle-aged, then elderly woman. He gave me a copy of something Dorothy had written for a college course that clearly showed her charming sense of humor. Listening, I heard his story as the love story it is, which is why John could be comfortable enough to shed some tears—sad, sweet, grateful tears. I didn't judge him for his human feelings of anger and resentment. He just told me about their life together and shared his tender and loving but also deeply sorrow-filled caregiving journey. I didn't try to "fix" him or change how he feels.

If you are a caregiver reading this chapter with countless mixed emotions and a grief process underway, like John you may need to let a family member or friend know that just listening is the best way to help. Be sure to choose someone unlikely to be judgmental. If necessary, you can explain that you're doing okay and that you don't need advice—just an opportunity to talk about things. It's how people heal.

NAOMI'S STORY

Guilt and Self-Forgiveness

When Naomi's dad was in the last months of his life, she thought he was "talking out of his head," but actually he wasn't. "Daddy kept telling me to write a check for $1,000 to my nephew, Jacob, who was getting married soon. He wanted to be sure to give his youngest grandson the same wedding gift he'd given grandsons Adam, David, and Barry."

"But Daddy, you *didn't* give checks that big to the other boys. You were generous, though, and gave them each $250," Naomi told him. She could see that her dad was upset. He argued with her about wanting to give the larger amount to equal things out, but Naomi thought he just wasn't thinking clearly anymore, perhaps due to all the medicines he was taking.

"I wrote out a check for $250 and he signed it but he wasn't happy about it. I knew Daddy had always bent over backwards to be fair and I was trying to help him be true to those values to the end of his life. I was also afraid that Jacob's older brother, Adam, would be hurt if Daddy gave Jacob a much larger wedding gift than Adam had received a few years earlier."

Naomi's father, Saul, always had been smart with numbers, careful about record keeping, frugal in saving for his and his wife's old age, yet generous in giving to his daughter, son, and grandsons. "Daddy was especially good at thinking about money," Naomi explained. "He still had these qualities at the end of his life but he didn't have the ability to communicate." Sadly, this is how Naomi missed her beloved dad's effort, before he died, to make things fair for his youngest grandson. "I just thought he was completely confused," Naomi told me.

After her father passed away, Naomi was cleaning out an old file cabinet in his apartment when she came across a piece of cardboard, the kind used by dry cleaners, folded within men's pressed shirts. Taped to the cardboard were five cancelled checks for $1,000 each—made out to Naomi, her brother Saul, and grandsons Adam, David, and Barry. There was no $1,000 cancelled check for Jacob! Her dad had been right to realize—but, in his frail condition, was unable to explain—that Jacob hadn't yet been born in 1981, when all those checks were written.

"Daddy had gotten a promotion at work," Naomi recalled, more than 30 years later. "I can just imagine how good it made him feel that he could give those gifts to his children and grandchildren." He saved the cancelled checks in such a sweet and special way, in a place kept safe until his dying days. That spring when Jacob was to graduate from medical school and get married the next day, his proud grandfather wanted to be sure this youngest grandson was remembered, honored properly and equally.

"For months, it hurt me so badly after I realized what I didn't know until it was too late. I struggled to forgive myself for not doing what Daddy told me to do, not understanding that he had a good reason for wanting me to write Jacob a $1,000 check. He just wanted Jacob to have the same gift that he'd given to everybody else. And I didn't give Daddy the pleasure of knowing that he'd done that."

Naomi was right that her dad *had* given $250 to the other grandsons for their weddings. And she was right to try to help him live by the same code of fairness she'd seen in her dad and respected throughout her life.

"I told my brother and we agreed to draw from our own inheritance and write a check to Jacob for $1,000 and explain to him that Daddy wanted him to have it. So we honored our father's last wish and I've had to forgive myself for what I didn't know.

"You do the best you can and that's all you can do as a caregiver," Naomi says. "And some days what you can do is not good enough and you have to be able to forgive yourself."

SOPHIA'S STORY

Sophia, like many daughters-in-law in Hispanic or Latino families, was expected to take on the primary responsibility for her husband's elderly parents' care. She was devoted to her husband, dearly loved his parents as if they were her own, and genuinely *wanted* to express her love for all three of them by helping out as much as possible. Several aspects of the caregiving situation over the years, however, were so exasperating and infuriating that Sophia felt horribly guilty for the anger she felt.

Calling them "Grandpa" and "Grandma," Sophia described driving her in-laws to their frequent doctor appointments. "Their physicians would often be late so sometimes we sat for hours in the waiting room, then the folks always wanted to go out to 'lunch' afterwards, whatever time it was. They'd fuss about which restaurant was best. It was like dealing with two kids. I called upon my child rearing skills, addressing these two 90-year-olds," Sophia explained. "Okay. Grandpa, you picked last time so now it's Grandma's turn." Especially frustrating was the fact that it would take either or both of them "forever" to make a decision.

"It was the same way at the grocery store," Sophia went on. "Grandma had so little control over Grandpa's illnesses, her blindness, and their inability to stay in their own apartment unless they had help that she wanted control over *something*. She had to have *exactly* what she wanted in the way of groceries. I had to read her all the labels until I finally named the right item, such as 'white, thin sliced Wonder Bread.' Only then would she finally let me put whatever it was in the cart she was pushing to steady herself."

Accusations of Stealing

As the couple's health failed further, Sophia and her husband knew it wasn't safe for the folks to stay alone in their apartment and moved them to semiassisted living. "Grandpa had lost so much of his strength," Sophia explained. "We knew he couldn't drive anymore so, after we tried unsuccessfully to get them to sell their car, we moved it to our house where there was room to park it."

The next time she went over to see them, Sophia was shocked to hear her father-in-law shout, "You guys stole our car! How dare you!" It was the first time he had ever even raised his voice to her in her 40 years of marriage to his son.

Sophia responded, "Grandpa, we didn't steal it! We aren't driving it. There just isn't a place to park it here without paying a lot of money every month."

"To be accused of stealing made me so angry, I could hardly see straight! I went home and told Antonio, 'It just feels so hurtful and insulting—when we are knocking ourselves out to be there for them every day and are taking good care of them!'

"It *is* very confusing to the caregiver," Sophia told me. "So often people go in and out of dementia. They're perfectly coherent, then 15 minutes later or the next day, they'll do or say something so off the wall that it makes you furious. It's hard not to get angry when they're flipping back and forth. It's hard to figure out what is dementia and what isn't.

"Meanwhile," Sophia lamented, "Grandma, who did *not* have dementia, could never seem to say, 'Thank you' or 'I'm sorry.' It would have meant the world to me if she'd just said, 'Thanks so much for all the help with grocery shopping.'"

After both of her in-laws were simultaneously hospitalized with pneumonia and returned home needing oxygen, they had home health care for a few weeks. "A few months later, after Grandpa was diagnosed with terminal cancer, he suffered a fall," Sophia remembers, "and after that he was bedridden. Grandma's blindness prevented her from taking care of Grandpa, so Antonio and I stayed with them 24/7, sleeping on the sofa bed in the living room. Grandpa was weak and would sleep all day, then wake up at 11:00 p.m. and yell because he wanted company. Antonio was still trying to work during the day, and Grandpa just wanted us to get up and visit with him. He was 'bored,' he said."

Sometime later, when the elderly man was near death, Sophia and Antonio's daughter was having surgery to remove a suspicious tumor everyone was worried about, so Antonio's sister came from out of state to stay with the folks. After two days, Sophia recalled, "Antonio's sister complained that taking care of them was 'really hard.' Since we had been taking care of them for *two years*, 'really hard' was an understatement! I used to just beg some of our family members to call and talk with them, but they mostly said it made them sad to hear how much Grandma and Grandpa were failing and they rarely called.

"After Grandpa died and I took even more care of Grandma," Sophia recalled, "I felt she was less and less appreciative, and more and more resentful of me. I began to resent Antonio even though he was very grateful for everything I was doing. I especially resented that Antonio was perfect in his mother's eyes and she was being so unkind to me.

"As a person ages and is more frail and dependent," Sophia realizes now, "they take out their resentment on whoever is simultaneously a 'safe target' and providing the most care.

"At one point when Grandma decided I was stealing from her because I paid her bills," Sophia remembers, "it was the last straw for me. My mother-in-law said, 'I don't want you writing checks anymore. Women can't deal with these things as well as men!' I left her apartment with steam coming out of my ears!"

Feeling Guilty for Feeling So Angry

Before and after her father-in-law's death, Sophia struggled fiercely with feelings of guilt. "I would feel worse sitting in church," she told me. "I loved them. I did. I loved Antonio's parents *so* much. But when both of them were still alive, I was becoming more resentful. The tension increased. I'd get mad and I'm not a person who gets mad easily.

"I cried almost every week when I went to Mass. I could hardly get through it for all the sadness and exhaustion that overwhelmed me. There were angry thoughts that I felt so bad for having. I'd go to confession and say, 'I love my mother-in-law but it's killing me!' I'd do penance, leave confession, and not feel better."

Lessons Learned

Now that eight years have passed since both of her husband's parents have been gone, Sophia says, "I'm really thankful Antonio's parents didn't have to go to a nursing home. I thank God for that."

Looking back, Sophia explains that finding humor in otherwise nerve-wracking situations *did* help mitigate some feelings of resentment. Once when she and Antonio were on a trip, "Grandma called 911 in the middle of the night and said she was having trouble breathing. Our daughter, Maria, met the ambulance and stayed with her grandmother while the emergency room doctors checked her out and couldn't find anything wrong. At 2:00 a.m., as they were leaving the hospital, Grandma said, 'I'm hungry. I want something to eat.' With some difficulty, Maria managed to locate a McDonald's restaurant that was open all night. As they drove home Grandma complained, 'Maria, when *your sister* takes me out to eat, *she* always takes me to Macaroni Grill!'

"Humor," Sophia continued, "sometimes is all that gets you through. We still tell that story and laugh about it." Sophia almost always eventually finds it within herself to thank God for the tension-breaking, resentment-reducing, stress-relieving gift of seeing humor in tough situations.

If she could go back in time to do something different to lighten her load, Sophia says, "I would take better care of myself." During those years of stress, "I tried to spend time with friends, went for walks as often as I could, did a few yoga classes for the arthritis in my knees and hips, and sometimes I even played some golf. But it wasn't enough."

In addition, if Sophia had it to do over again, "I would be more assertive with Antonio's relatives, and even to long-term friends, about how something as simple as a ten minute phone call could make Grandma's day. I wouldn't say it when I was angry, and I'd say it in a loving way, in a moment when I was in control. But I'd let them know that 'even if it is frustrating for you to wait for the phone to ring several times until Grandma can pick up, or even if you do have a busy day, ten minutes is not too much to give to Grandma to bring her a tiny bit of joy.'"

When other family members say it makes them sad to call or come visit the loved one for whom you are the primary caregiver, it is important not to "guilt trip" them, which is how Sophia's words above might have been heard had she spoken them. I recommend simply being honest about the stress and sadness *you* are experiencing: "I get pretty worn out caring for Grandma mostly on my own," Sophia might have said. "I really need you to call her regularly and visit us—you will lift her spirits and mine, too!"

After Antonio's parents died, Sophia called her own sister, brother, and sister-in-law in New Mexico to thank them for the "amazingly loyal and selfless care" they had provided for *their* mother. "I apologized for *my own inability to cope* and my arrogance in not realizing how hard it was on my sister, brother, and his wife that I left *them* with the care of *our* mother—who lived in my brother's home for six years and then lingered bedridden in a nursing home for the last two years, unable to speak or recognize anyone."

Being a caregiver offers one lesson after another in humility: We don't get through this life very successfully without learning to accept our human limitations and weaknesses. While learning to forgive others' failings and our own, it is equally important to show ourselves some kindness and give ourselves credit for having done the best that we could at the time. As we age ourselves, Sophia says, we recognize that WE will be the ones needing care from our own children in the not too distant future.

SUSAN'S STORY

In almost every family, the responsibility for elder parent caregiving falls primarily to one family member, usually a daughter and often the oldest child. Patterns set in childhood and adolescence as to what is expected of each family member typically reemerge as we get older, but in some cases last a lifetime. The helping roles we play through the years that enrich our lives with purpose, value, and joy also give rise to resentment when what we give to our loved ones is simply expected and taken for granted or goes unappreciated.

Susan's caregiving role dates back to childhood. She was 11 years old when she started babysitting her younger sisters, who were 9 and 3. At 13, her mother—described by Susan as "not Miss Maternal"—relied on her to babysit those two plus a new baby sister.

When riots broke out in Newark and elsewhere around the country in 1968 following the assassination of Martin Luther King Jr., her mother told Susan to leave Rutgers University after her first year of college. Saying Susan would be "safer" at home, even though her university was nowhere near a troubled city, offered Susan's mother an odd but convenient excuse to have the 18-year-old's continuing help with the youngest sister, who was five. Susan commuted from home in rural Delaware to attend a less prestigious local college and never went back to Rutgers, despite having earned her place there with hard work and a strong academic record.

At 19, Susan married and moved away from home. She quit school, became a mother, divorced, finished college, and launched a teaching career while raising her daughter as a single parent. For the better part of three decades, Susan's caregiving focused on being a loving mom and a dedicated, fun-loving kindergarten teacher. There were big family gatherings at her parents' house every holiday and always on Sunday nights.

At 49, long since happily remarried, Susan left her rewarding work in early childhood education to become a family caregiver once again. Her elderly mother's memory and eyesight were failing, and one of her sisters needed help with a newly adopted baby. Her other two sisters had busy lives of their own and looked to Susan to bear the burden as she always had. In addition, Susan's daughter was expecting her first child. Susan was looking forward to supporting her daughter and to becoming a grandmother.

Susan, helping out at her parents' house, began to find "way old food" in their refrigerator and saw her dad upset that "the house was in disarray." The combination of her mom's macular degeneration, forgetfulness, and trouble doing her usual household jobs made Susan realize, "This is not my mother because everything used to be spotless."

Dealing with Your Elderly Loved One's Loss of Control

When her mother was a young woman, she taught piano lessons and was the vice principal of an elementary school, then for many years directed the choir and played the organ at their church. She must have found it very difficult to cope with her ever-worsening impairments. "Mom resented me big time as she started to decline and all the way up to her death," Susan vividly recalls.

Susan was coming more and more often to help out at the house. Even knowing that they couldn't manage without their oldest daughter's help, her mother would say, "I don't want you here!"

It was hard for a loving daughter to hear such hurtful words, but she relied a lot on the "great advice" she got from the Alzheimer's Association. Susan would say, "Oh, Mom, *you* could do all of this housework if it weren't for the trouble with your eyesight." Then her mom would let her help, especially with laundry and changing linens. "At other times, I would fib a little," Susan went on. "I'd tell her, 'I just can't sit still and, besides, this sorting and cleaning is fun for me.'"

Growing old and needing other people's help to manage one's daily life leads to losing control. Feeling vulnerable in so many ways, it is pretty understandable if the person you are caring for sometimes feels resentful. Rather than getting defensive, Susan told me that she chose not to respond in any direct way to her mother's anger. "I learned pretty quickly to work around Mom, not to tell her exactly what I was doing. *Also I did not challenge her if she wanted me to stop.* Many times, if she was napping, I would hurry and clean out the old food or finish the housework." Susan had the right idea.

In late adulthood, people often feel they are being treated with condescension, as if once again a child. Not infrequently, the elderly respond in anger because they *are* being treated like children by their family members or paid caregivers. For this reason, the insights of child psychologist Haim Ginott are fitting here. "Dependency breeds hostility," he said, in a public lecture I attended. It made such an impression on me that I remember Dr. Ginott's words more than 40 years later.

"Ladies and gentlemen, children are not our friends," continued Dr. Ginott. "Children are our enemies!" On hearing this, the several hundred moms and dads in attendance broke into laughter and applause. I myself was not yet a parent and I didn't understand why the audience was roaring. "Children are our enemies," he went on, "because children are dependent on us. Therefore, reduce dependency and you will reduce the hostility."

Dr. Ginott was talking to parents about children needing choices in order to become more capable of doing things for themselves. Good feelings replace resentment when a child is given more independence and grows in self-efficacy. Dr. Ginott's lesson is similarly applicable to the elderly person whose increasing disabilities in old age often shatter a lifetime of hard won autonomy, dignity, and self-respect. No one wants to feel useless, and no one wants to return to being treated like a child.

To the greatest extent possible, the impaired loved one or nursing home resident needs to be regarded by family members and paid caregivers as an adult deserving of participation in decision making and daily activities. Whether it is being patient with the person who moves slowly so he can dress himself or she can walk with a cane instead of riding in a wheelchair, maintaining independence and mobility matters greatly. In nursing homes, it is especially offensive to me to see so many people kept in wheelchairs all day long, for the convenience of the nursing aides, and to see the televisions tuned to what the paid caregiver wants to watch, instead of something more likely to appeal to a patient with dementia, such as reruns of decades-old family sitcoms or children's programs.

Whether it is giving the elderly person a choice of what to have for lunch, asking for advice, or seeking help with folding the tea towels and washcloths, *reducing dependency and feelings of uselessness are effective ways to respond to the impaired person's feelings of resentment*. Susan did her parents' yard work while her dad supervised and helped as much as he was able. Her folks enjoyed their weekly outings to the grocery store because she let them make their own selections. Using her side vision, Susan's mom picked out the fruits and vegetables, as she had done for more than 50 years. "Dad would ride a scooter because of his vascular problems," Susan told me, and he went after the deli meats. "I saw that he was starting to forget things, but my parents always bought the exact same groceries so that wasn't a problem."

The Problem with Putting Others' Needs Ahead of Your Own

When isolation increases, the dementia often accelerates at a more rapid rate. "Now that mom couldn't see," Susan remembered, "she couldn't read or drive so she didn't want to go to Bingo. She quit her social groups and withdrew from the Ladies of Charity fund-raisers at church." Susan's dad, during this time, was a loving caregiver for his wife and was endeavoring to "cover for her memory problems." But Susan could see that her mom's decline was "wearing on his heart."

In 2001, Susan was by his side when her 83-year-old dad insisted on taking down a curtain rod, may have had a ministroke, fell, and broke his hip. Adding truth to the adage that "if things can get worse they probably will," while in the hospital her dad had a heart attack and had to have open-heart surgery. Her mom, Susan explained, "was 80 then, already in bad shape and repeating herself all the time, but still recognized people and knew where she was." Every day, Susan drove 45 minutes to her parents' house to get her mother, another 45 minutes to the hospital where she and her mother stayed the day. She did the reverse trips to take her mother home at night "when mom could still spend the night alone," then Susan went home to her husband. Remarkably, "Dad recovered enough to take over some of Mom's caregiving."

As mentioned earlier, the caregiving role in families often comes around like the proverbial brass ring on a merry-go-round. People who learned early to put others' needs and well-being before their own grab hold of the brass ring quite naturally. In Susan's family, she was always the one. By 2002, 53-year-old Susan spent three days a week babysitting two grandsons and two nephews at their three different homes. She often drove first to her parents' or daughter's house to help out and then to babysit for one of her sisters. Each family lived from 35 minutes to an hour away by car from Susan's home.

"You're not working. You have the time," is how one of the sisters rationalized the fact that Susan was doing almost all of her parents' caregiving and the other three sisters almost none. Such rationalization often results from feelings of guilt, when a family member *knows* she is not helping to carry an appropriate share of the load. What a difference it would have made had that sister said instead, "I know you are knocking yourself out to help Mom and Dad. It must be so exhausting. I wish I could help more. I *really* appreciate what you're doing, Susan, on behalf of all of us girls."

Susan loved her grandsons and fell in love with her nephews, too. She was also sympathetic to the fact that her sisters were each at a different place in their lives and less able to provide assistance to their parents. Because of the close relationship with their dad that Susan had, love motivated Susan to protect him and assist their folks in virtually every possible way.

The time came when "Dad would take a nap and Mom would get up and roam the neighborhood," Susan explained. "My parents were bad off and Dad decided they should move to an assisted living place. Within just three or four months, Mom needed to be in the Alzheimer's wing and Dad wanted to be with her, even though he didn't belong there. Dad found the place depressing. It was Nightmare City for him."

Feelings of Resentment and Sadness

It was not long until both parents needed a nursing home. Susan's three sisters insisted that the parents move to a facility near *their* homes, even though this particular place was located an hour away from Susan and her husband, Ben, who were the frail parents' only frequent visitors. "Ben loved my parents to death and he was generous in giving them companionship." It troubled Susan that her three sisters visited the nursing home only occasionally and the grandchildren never came. The grandkids all said they "wanted to remember Mom-Mom and PopPop as they were in the good days."

"It's too hard for me to see them this way" is a genuinely felt but frequent excuse given by family members who rationalize leaving the caregiving to others, as if the primary caregiver himself or herself doesn't find the whole thing excruciatingly painful, too, but nevertheless faithfully visits.

In 2007, "when Dad got pneumonia and died, Mom never knew it," Susan recalled. "In a way she was blessed because she never knew the pain of losing him. She'd ask where he was and I'd tell her that he was in the bedroom and she'd smile. If a man sat near her wheelchair at the group dining table, she'd assume it was Dad.

"There was scads of paperwork after Dad died and endless phone calls involving being put on hold for half an hour or more. One of my sisters and I had to handle the estate and Mom's finances and there was a lot of confusion."

Susan's sister said, "I can't do this. I can't stay on the phone forever!"

"And all that got dumped on me, even though I was grieving the hardest," Susan recalled, finally allowing herself to complain to me. It fell to Susan to "stay on the phone forever," waiting to get the legal and medical information necessary for her mother's ongoing care.

Susan was upset for over a year after her dad died. She recalls, "I was the crier. I was able to function, but I wanted to talk about him. My sisters just said, 'Oh, he's happy now, he's in Heaven.' But I *missed* him."

"Exactly a year after Dad died, I went to the Jersey Shore by myself, stayed in a little condo, and went to church every morning. I found great solace in that church, absolute peace. I said the rosary a couple of times. Once when I was sitting there praying and crying, a strange lady came up to me, never said a word, and gave me a hug.

"I walked the beach every day and I wrote letters to my dad in a journal. 'Show me a sign that you're there, Dad,' I said, and I asked him for a pretty seashell. On the last day walking on the beach, I found three special shells and I was sure he was there with me."

The following year, again on the anniversary of her dad's death, Susan went to the Shore again. "The year after, I felt I didn't need to do that. I was better. Not all the way, though."

Looking back, Susan understandably resents the fact that so much was expected of her and that her sisters gave so little help to their parents. Probably because they felt sheepish about taking advantage of Susan's good heart and willingness to shoulder most of the caregiving, rarely did the siblings ever think to thank her. One of Susan's sisters, in her own defense, put it this way, "You always did so we felt we didn't have to." Another sister excused herself by telling Susan, "You take on more than you can chew and then you resent that you had to do it."

These lingering remnants of resentment, however, are not something that Susan allows to alter the separate and unique sisterly bond she shares with Debby, Diane, and Laura. "My sisters are my best friends," she confidently declares. "Each is different, and I know which sister is the one to talk with, with which kind of problem, whenever I want to vent."

The Caregiver's Reward

Susan also realizes that her enduring reward for those long years of caregiving is the special closeness she shared with her dad. "I was Daddy's little girl to the nth degree and I was protecting him." His loving presence experienced at the beach a year after his death continues to be felt, warms Susan's heart, and comforts her still, eight years since his passing.

Susan fondly remembers all the times her dad thanked her. "He'd hug me over and over and say, 'You are so smart. You can handle everything. I'd never have lasted this long without you girls, including Mom.'" Susan recalls that he thanked them all but realizes that—because of all those years of caregiving—she is blessed beyond her sisters with a far more lasting and vivid experience of her dad's gratitude. She also carries no guilt, an emotional burden her sisters carry.

Finding Strength, Learning Self-Care

Sadly, Susan's mother, who had to be showered, dressed, fed, and pushed in her wheelchair at the nursing home, "lived for six more years, the last three of which she was bedridden." Susan visited her once or twice a week. "It got to the point of being painful," she told me. "You'd sit there. She didn't know you. The nursing home staff made jokes, but nothing was funny anymore. I really resented how the aides seemed to be laughing at the frail, sad people behind their backs, when a woman was crying or a man was walking around without his pants on. They were trying to make light of a situation, and I felt like I was dying of sadness."

Hopefully the aides weren't really making fun of their patients! Myself, having taught police officers, funeral directors, and physicians, I understand that "gallows humor" is sometimes used to mitigate the high stress of working daily in grim situations. I can only imagine the similarly stressful life of the aides who feed, bathe, dress, and change the diapers of frail elderly persons—aides working long hours in nursing homes, earning low wages. They should be trained to watch how they behave with the residents and their family members, however, so as not to use dark humor as a coping mechanism except in private. Frail elders and their loved ones deserve to be treated with respect and dignity.

As many of us do in the face of a loved one's unrelenting, incurable suffering or utter loss of dignity and quality of life, Susan hoped that her mother could just die in peace. "I prayed to God for years to just let her go. My mother was *gone* for so long before she died."

I wondered where Susan found the strength to be the adult child who was her parents' primary caregiver during the 15 years between the onset of her mother's impairments of vision and memory, through the decline of both parents, her dad's death, and the sad state of her mother having lingered so long without any quality of life until her death in 2013.

Most of all, Susan's 30-year relationship with her husband has been an abiding strength. "My parents loved Ben. They adopted him and he them. And Ben was a very good listener, empathic, and very helpful especially to *me* during all those difficult years." She told me, "He just plain loved and admired my parents as much as his own . . . and Ben is a very loving, giving man." He didn't feel like he was sacrificing. He worried about the stress she was under and was happy to help.

The rituals and hymns of her church since childhood "more than anything" gave and continue to give Susan sustenance. "I say prayers over Dad and everything else lately," she says. "I have so much to be grateful for. I was a Catholic school teacher for 18 years and it's a huge part of who I am."

For the past 15 years, Susan has gone to the same chiropractor for treatments to combat neck and back pain that had its onset and got its momentum from the physical labor and emotional stress of providing caregiving for so many family members. "I'd end up crying when the doctor worked on me. He'd say, 'What is it today?' And I'd tell him about my dad or mother and whatever problem we were dealing with at the time. The doctor listened and always gave me a hug before I left his office. 'You're good to go now,' he'd say. 'You'll be okay. Go get 'em!'"

It was helpful, during the hardest caregiving years, to commiserate by phone with an old friend who was taking care of her frail elderly parents, too. Every few months she shared and still shares good times with five special girlfriends. "We can talk for hours and hours." Susan also stays in touch with several teacher friends who were colleagues for many years. These days, as always, Susan and Ben stay close to their three grandsons, nephews, and niece. She goes dog-walking-while-talking several times a week with her girlfriends.

"But I'm still not good at taking care of myself," Susan says. By this she means that it's hard to say no to family members when asked for help, even when it's inconvenient or her chronic neck pain and back spasms are bothering her.

There is a wider meaning in Susan's realization that "I'm not good at taking care of myself." It is a common problem for those of us who have shaped our identity and overly defined our self-worth by the good that we do for others. Often we feel we have value *only* because we work hard and devote our energies to helping people in need.

Susan's life is precious, and her worth as a person is profound simply because of the person she *is*. She needs to learn—as do many of us—that we are valuable just as we are. Our lives matter even when we sometimes say no to the people we care about in order to take care of ourselves.

TO REDUCE FEELINGS OF RESENTMENT, BUDGET YOUR "EMOTIONAL HOSPITALITY"

During the 10 years when I was teaching young doctors while on the faculty of a family practice residency program, I saw in some of the resident physicians a considerable amount of resentment. Most of them complained to their colleagues in private, but one young man had to be reprimanded for unprofessional, unethical behavior when he yelled at a patient, "If you don't stop smoking, I'm going to stop writing these prescriptions for your high blood pressure medicine!" His behavior, of course, was the exception, and he was given direction and more closely supervised thereafter.

Most of these sleep-deprived, hardworking, dedicated young physicians had a caring demeanor and an idealism I admired. They had chosen family medicine over specialty areas that would earn them far more over a lifetime. Still, many seemed surprised and some said they felt angry when their sick patients didn't take their medicine or otherwise failed to comply with "doctor's orders." I talked with these conscientious men and women, recently out of medical school, about the concept of emotional hospitality.

"It's wonderful that you care so much about your patients, go the extra mile with them and are generous in how much time you devote to each individual. But the fact that you are constantly fatigued and overloaded with responsibilities makes you vulnerable to getting cynical early in your career or (worse) puts you at risk of losing your temper."

I then shared with the residents something I was taught in my own training as a therapist: "If I care more about my patients' well-being and work harder to solve their problems than *they* themselves do, I'm going to feel resentful. Furthermore, if I find myself becoming irritated and impatient with or judgmental of the individual who I'm trying to help, this is a clear signal that I'm not taking good enough care of *myself*."

It is the same for personal caregivers. For example, if you are caring for your mother and she is unable to help herself in many or most ways, you may need to ask other family members for help or hire paid caregivers for respite and support. When so much of your time is not your own, you must set aside some time that routinely becomes solely your own.

What emotional hospitality is about is "touching" another person with empathy, active listening, kindness, and helpfulness. Most of us aspire to be good people, able in these ways to make a difference in the lives of those we care about. Because we're human beings and not saints, however, we can't always be "on" or always giving. Resentment can result when we expect too much of ourselves and neglect our own physical or mental health.

There must be time, intentionally planned-for time, for *all* caregivers to nurture themselves. Being a family caregiver of an impaired elderly loved one can be just as stressful as being a stretched thin, highly fatigued family doctor with a waiting room full of sick patients.

How will *you* take care of yourself, make arrangements for the time away from caregiving that is needed to sustain your energy, reduce feelings of resentment, and allow for the recreational activities, exercise, relaxation, and time alone that all caregivers need? Start now to think about this question and find the answers that are best for you.

Caregiver Stress—What Helps and What Usually Doesn't

So no matter what the demands on your time right now, take a step back. Breathe deeply and slowly. Get some perspective. And tend to yourself. Oddly enough, it will help you be a calmer, gentler, and more efficient caregiver.

—Virginia Morris, elder care authority and author,
How to Care for Aging Parents

Caregiving is hard work. Whether you live in another state or city, across town or share the same home, taking care of an impaired elderly loved can be a draining experience. Being stretched to the limits of your energy, patience, problem-solving abilities, and good intentions, at times you may feel almost desperate for relief. Even under the best of circumstances—when providing care for an elderly loved one who expresses gratitude and manages to keep a remarkably positive attitude—still, there are plenty of challenges. It is especially hard to cope when you're feeling fatigued.

The greater the physical and (especially) the mental disabilities of the loved one you're caring for, the more apt you are to feel burdened, unless you employ some of the stress buffering strategies known to be effective for replenishing your energy and lifting your spirits. Even if your family member isn't yet (or won't become) severely cognitively impaired, you're probably looking for ways to surmount some significant challenges.

THE STRESS OF CARING FOR A FAMILY MEMBER
WITH MILD COGNITIVE IMPAIRMENTS

Observing the onset of what researchers call mild cognitive impairment (MCI) in your spouse, parent, or other relative can be distressing. You don't know what is causing the behavioral changes you're seeing, and you don't know what will happen next. Doctors may be able to rule out or treat related medical problems, but often they can't give you a definitive diagnosis or prognosis to alleviate your worry and anxiety.

In their study of responses to the onset of MCI, Rosemary Blieszner and Karen Roberto found that "even in this early caregiving stage . . . some care partners are quite distressed by the behavioral changes they are observing in the older adult with MCI. In addition, not only was their relationship with [their loved one] changed, many also felt isolated from their larger social network."[1]

If you find yourself in this situation, you may not feel free to leave your loved one alone and take a break to do what you enjoy. You may hesitate to ask others for help because you're worried that things might get worse down the road and *then* you'll need to ask for help. As a result, you increase your risk of depression and the irritability, impaired concentration, fatigue, sadness, and low self-esteem that come with it. What's more, if you find yourself becoming impatient or feeling angry with your loved one, you may begin to feel that you are not the kind, caring person you want to be. How you perceive the changes in your loved one with MCI, and how burdened you feel by the demands on your time and your new responsibilities, will likely determine how much distress and anxiety you feel.[2] Thankfully there are self-care strategies that can help you cope with the inevitable stress. Below I list and comment on strategies that Blieszner and Roberto suggest:

- "Learn not to blame yourself." Part of simply being human is having times of feeling impatient, angry, and at a loss as to how to respond to these new challenges.
- "Strengthen your coping skills." You can learn to handle strong emotions and frustrating situations, in the ways this chapter will discuss in great detail.
- "Take care of your own health." Sleep; exercise; friendships; moderation in food and drink; well visits for preventive care from your dentist, family physician or internist, or gynecologist; and keeping up with vaccinations— all are ways to keep yourself mentally and physically strong.

- "Seek and accept respite." Reach out for and let yourself receive support from others, including from individuals and community agencies.
- "Take time for yourself." Time away from caregiving, even for short periods at a time, promotes "psychological well-being." Small ways to renew yourself matter, such as taking walks, sitting in a coffee shop or on a park bench with a newspaper or crossword puzzle, and enjoying a phone visit with a friend.
- "Learn to communicate more effectively with your loved one with MCI and significant others." It never helps to argue but almost always is helpful to listen, ask questions to clarify what the other person is saying, and acknowledge the other person's feelings as worthy of being heard.
- "Make good use of any spiritual or religious resources you find meaningful, including meditation, prayer, or rituals of faith." Studies show that "those who value religion [and] employ religious coping," have a significant resource for strength that also has been shown to be effective.[3]

Absolutely every one of these strategies applies equally well to taking care of a loved one with a major neurocognitive disorder (major NCD), Alzheimer's disease, Lewy bodies, vascular disorders, Parkinson's disease, or another medical condition. Whatever the cause, dementia is often accompanied by problems that are devastatingly complex by nature, and physically draining and emotionally exhausting for the family caregiver.

Your first challenge may be to realize that, *through no choice or fault of their own, many people in late adult life pose an endless set of challenges for their caregivers.* The ravages of dementia or severe physical disabilities may have changed the person you love into someone quite different. As a caregiver, you will need to develop an ever-changing set of skills to cope with these new problem behaviors and, at the same time, take care of your own needs. It's sad to see these changes in the person you care so much about. If he or she is ordering you around like a servant or being verbally abusive, you probably feel some anger as well as sadness. You need effective strategies to help calm your elderly loved one and manage your own emotions.

DEALING WITH A DIFFICULT, DEPENDENT PERSON

Some people become difficult and demanding in their old age, changing from the loving people they were. Other people have always had troublesome personalities and troubled relationships, making the impairments of aging and the usual challenges of caregiving even more complicated. You probably need a quiverful of new arrows to fire at all the problems you're trying to solve. Dealing with a person who has strained your capacity to cope with him or her for much of your life requires planning ahead, rehearsing your choice of words, and finding new ways of providing care.

LILLIAN'S DAD

Certainly this was true for Lillian, whose father was remarkably difficult. Even though she had never gotten along with her father and had long been the target of his harsh and hurtful words, she visited the 95-year-old widower almost daily and faithfully oversaw his care in a nursing facility near her home. When Lillian told him that his son had cancer, her sibling just a year younger, the old man's immediate response was, "Well, if George dies, you can't go to the funeral! You have to stay in town to take care of *me*!" Even though this uncaring response was typical of her father, hearing those words applied to her *brother* shocked this 70-year-old daughter to her core. Lillian stared at him cold faced, long enough for him to notice, then left the room in silence. Not responding in anger but walking away took great restraint but is an effective way to answer such a perennially selfish parent. This was a man destined to put his own well-being ahead of all others—all the way to his grave—she realized.

Later, Lillian would share her feelings of dismay and outrage with her sister and daughter but not with her brother, of course. She knew that arguing with her father would accomplish nothing and that his pleas would never keep her from visiting her brother during his battle with cancer or attending his funeral if he passed away, regardless of his living in a state far away.

In 71 years of marriage, this was a widower whose ever-present wife had catered to his every need and demand, like many women who promised to "love and obey" their husbands. Now he feared being left alone, despite living in a home-like facility where his caregiver had only two other frail elders to look after. Lillian's other way of coping when he said something unkind, racist, homophobic, or ridiculously demanding was to respond briefly before changing the subject, "Daddy, stop that!" or, matter-of-factly, "Daddy, you know that's [untrue, unkind, unfair]." After that, saying in a calm tone of voice that she was going out to take a walk seemed to drive home the message that such conversations or topics would not be engaged.

Whether your loved one was easy to get along with but has become difficult and demanding in old age or has always seemed self-absorbed, there are problem-solving skills that can significantly reduce your caregiver stress. Empowering yourself to respond with both firmness and kindness to your impaired, increasingly dependent family member is one of the best things you can do to help yourself *and* your loved one.

Lillian's short story shows us how she did that, as does Janet's much longer story that follows, with many ins and outs involving three siblings and a demanding parent.

JANET, DANIEL, AND MYRA'S MOTHER

To help me understand the caregiving challenges she and her siblings still have with their mother, Janet wanted to explain the 89-year-old's long history of giving commands and expecting deferential compliance from family members, household employees, and her students. Demonstrating the adage that our greatest strengths often are the flip side of our most noteworthy weaknesses, Mrs. Duncan's gumption and strong-willed personality led to many accomplishments, while her stubbornness and sense of entitlement made her difficult to deal with over the years.

Born in 1926 into a well-to-do family, Mrs. Duncan enjoyed privileges of comfort and social status, including growing up with a maid and gardener who served the family. The man she married, also born in 1926, rose to become a highly successful bank executive and continued to provide her with the amenities to which she had become accustomed, including membership in the local country club. Keeping up appearances was very important to Mrs. Duncan in ways Janet, Daniel, and Myra sometimes found hurtful as children and still find hard to cope with as adults.

"A typical example from when we were growing up," Janet explained, "is that my sister didn't get along with our mother. Myra was a little girl who never wanted to wear dresses and was constantly battling to march to her own drummer. When I was 14 and she was 4, it would take forever for all of us to get in the car to go someplace because of the endless arguments over Myra wanting to wear pants."

"I don't want my friends to see my daughter wearing trousers," Mrs. Duncan would say. "Myra, go change your clothes!"

"Mom, let her wear pants!" Janet, now age 64, recalls saying to their mother again and again. As her parents' firstborn, Janet often played a conciliatory, leadership role in the family.

"Finally, I just told my little sister *not* to change into a dress, and I said to our mother, 'Mom, we'll be in the car and ready to leave when you are.'

"As the years passed," Janet continued, "Myra was never given any credit for her accomplishments, never seemed to be the person Mom wanted her to be. She left home for college, moved far away, and bought a farm with her long-time partner."

When both Myra and Daniel came out to their parents at the ages of 25 and 30, Janet remembers, "My mother said, 'Don't tell your kids!' And I said, 'Mom, Myra and Daniel are kind, loving people. They're just gay, get over it!' And eventually she did."

At the age of 50, Mrs. Duncan had gone back to college to earn a master's degree in special education. She taught children with dyslexia for 20 years, then tutored young people with disabilities past her seventy-eighth birthday. Having long been an independent-minded, intelligent, capable person living an active life, understandably, made it extra hard for Mrs. Duncan to accept advice from her adult children once she was a widow showing early signs of dementia.

The three siblings were overruled when they urged their mother to choose an independent living community with assisted living and nursing care available down the road should it be needed. Janet, taking the lead in facilitating her mother's care, had tried unsuccessfully to talk her mother into a highly desirable local facility with multiple levels of care. It was a very nice place that would have guaranteed the ability to stay even if her mother's life savings ran out after the required $280,000 deposit and she was eventually no longer able to pay rent.

Instead, Mrs. Duncan, at 85, chose an equally lovely senior living facility without the availability of advanced care. Here, should she run out of money and her comparable initial deposit becomes depleted, she is not protected from having to move to another facility affordable only through public assistance (Medicaid). Like the facility she rejected, Mrs. Duncan's independent living apartment complex has several restaurants, an exercise room, hair salon, movie theater, pool, and an auditorium for special events. A staff member at the facility comes to clean her apartment once a week, changes the sheets every other week, and someone is always on hand to make needed plumbing or appliance repairs. All residents are provided with an iPad for the purpose of checking in daily. If they've not been heard from by 10 a.m., someone will come to the door to check on them.

Expecting Too Much from Paid Helpers

As Mrs. Duncan's dementia has advanced, however, she needs companionship and oversight to help with her medicines, meals, shopping, and transportation. So, to look after her mother on the days when no family member was available, Janet hired a companion through an agency. "She was a nice African American lady, but I was appalled when I got a call from my mother," Janet recalls.

"I know you're at the office," Mrs. Duncan said to her elder daughter, "but we have a little problem. This woman doesn't seem to want to iron my clothes."

"Mom," Janet exclaimed, "she is not your maid!"

"Here was a kind-hearted person working for an agency," Janet told me, "who was probably only getting $12 from the $18 an hour we were paying the agency. I felt disgusted over my mother's attitude and went over there to tell her so."

"Oh, I didn't do anything wrong," Mrs. Duncan told Janet. "I treated her fine."

For the next month, Janet tried to right the situation, but "there was no changing my mother's attitude because it went back 80 years. She was treating this black woman like her servant, ordering her to do all sorts of things like cleaning the stove."

Janet felt she couldn't let this good person keep working for their family. "I told the woman, 'I'm not going to have you subjected to this! If my mother can't treat you right, she's not going to have you.'

"Please accept my apology for my mother's behavior," Janet continued. "She grew up on a farm with no experience of African Americans except their employees and that's all she knows."

The 40-year-old woman sent by the agency to be a companion care provider was gracious in her reply. "I understand," she said.

Janet then hired one of her daughter's friends, a trained geriatric aide, "who Mother immediately put to work polishing her silver and *that* lasted a month. Then we tried a white lady from the same agency the black lady came from. She lasted three months until she also got sick of my mother treating her like a servant."

Whether self-employed or hired by agencies to work in independent and assisted living situations or nursing homes, elder companions and nursing aides commonly are poorly paid. Many are members of minority populations who for cultural, religious, and financial reasons are unlikely to employ others to take care of their own elderly family members. Whether they are African Americans, Hispanic Americans, Asian Americans, or Middle Eastern Americans or come from white working-class families, it is probably not an overstatement to say that a majority of these caregivers are barely earning enough to support their own families.

Family members who hire companions or care providers need to have job descriptions spelled out in writing, agreed upon in advance, and adhered to with mutual respect. To her credit, Janet communicated honestly and interacted respectfully with each of the women who provided support to her mother. Knowing how difficult it was for paid helpers not to be manipulated into doing work beyond what was appropriate, Janet was beginning to realize that it was time to make other arrangements for her mother's care.

You Still Have a Lot of Life to Live

Janet's husband saw that his wife—also barraged with unreasonable demands—thus far was being outmaneuvered by her mother. Several times a day, his mother-in-law was calling Janet at her office, interrupting meetings with clients and expecting an immediate response to the elderly woman's seemingly constant medical and other complaints. On one occasion, Mrs. Duncan, bleeding from a Band-Aid she'd just removed, called Janet to say, "You have to come right now!" This was a typically anxious and "urgent" medical plea made unnecessary by the fact that a nurse was on duty around the clock at the assisted living facility, only one floor down from her mother's apartment. Janet was often leaving work to run over to her mother's place in such nonemergency situations.

"I can see how she's manipulating you," Janet's husband said. "This is not right! You still have a lot of life to live and need to learn to deal with her so she doesn't run you ragged." Clearly a solution had to be found to address the problem of Mrs. Duncan's habitually demanding and manipulative behaviors. Caregiver stress overload was taking its toll on his wife in ways long obvious to the family. Fortunately, and to the benefit of her own physical and mental health, Janet listened to her husband.

What the research tells us is that *problem solving* is the best coping strategy for reducing stress and distress. Formulating and implementing "a plan of action to address the source of a problem" has been shown in studies by elder care medical experts JoAnn Tschanz and colleagues, to "foster personal growth and may help caregivers experience meaning in their roles," strengthening the caregiver's ability to cope with "the challenges presented by the care recipient's condition."[4] By coming up with the care-providing plan Janet described to me, she and her siblings (for the most part) have been able to stop resenting their mother and are able to "grow as persons in a good way."[5]

Because they were at the impressionable ages of 24, 15, and 12 when their mother went back to college at age 50, despite their father's "not being wild about it," the siblings saw her then as a strong, resourceful woman. Teaching and tutoring special education children for more than 25 years demonstrated a "can-do" approach to life that makes her still a positive role model for her children. "Although she was hovering and overbearing," Janet explains, giving credit to her mother where it's well deserved, "we can *respect* her for making *us* problem solvers, giving us the tools to figure out things like this."

Considering the alternatives, Janet, Daniel, and Myra decided and all agreed that Daniel would become their mother's primary caregiver. He would be paid a salary from their mother's savings, enabling him to leave the job with which he'd been unhappy for quite some time.

Daniel now earns his living by coming to her apartment and taking care of their mother four days a week. "She is sleepy and not yet alert when Daniel gets there," Janet explains. "He fixes her breakfast, gives her medicines, lays out her clothes, then tells her to shower and dress herself. He makes calls and pays her bills online while she's in the shower, and on some days he goes to the grocery store and returns quickly. Daniel does the laundry, cleaning, and cooking, drives his mother to her medical appointments and to the salon to get her hair done or for manicures, and pedicures when needed, and sometimes they go out to lunch."

The other three days, Janet does her part in sharing caregiving tasks. The siblings also hire a woman to help out one or two days a week or pay a friend of Daniel's who works with disabled adults. Myra occasionally comes from out of state to spend a week or two in her mother's apartment, when asked to give Daniel respite. Recently when Janet was out of state for a grandson's birthday celebration, Daniel and Myra met with a neurologist and social worker to discuss their mother's recent brain scan and the state of her health. "The three of us are so lucky," Janet told me, "that we're all on the same page, all help each other."

Creating Needed Boundaries

For a time his mother was so demanding that Daniel felt overwhelmed and emotionally exhausted. After looking after her needs for five or more hours, Daniel would be gone from her apartment barely a few minutes when she would call his cell phone to say tearfully, "I'm lonely!"

As happens, whether purposefully and intentionally or unconsciously, impaired elders who control so little in their lives often become demanding and manipulative, explains Virginia Morris, a nationally recognized authority on elder care. In *How to Care for Aging Parents*, Morris writes, "Complaining, calling constantly, or becoming sick at just the wrong moment can be an effective way to control other people. Your parent gripes, and you come running or cancel your vacation."[6]

"I told Daniel," Janet continued, "over the next year you're going to say, 'Oh, my mother's personality has changed.' It will seem different but it's the same. Dad just used to cushion it for us sibs because he did whatever she wanted."

Janet also told her brother, "Daniel, you need to say to Mom, 'I'm sorry you feel this way. I understand you're not happy. But if you continue this behavior, I will not be able to take care of you because I will get burned out.'"

"It worked immediately," Janet told me. "She has not called him crying anymore."

Janet, who is a financial planner, says that in dealing with clients for 20 years, "I've learned through experience how to handle people. You have to be kind, firm, factual, and not emotional. You can't let your emotions get away from you."

Virginia Morris, a very helpful writer I quoted at the opening of this chapter, uses bold print when she tells caregivers, "**Avoid Manipulation**." She goes on to say how to do this: "Set firm, clear limits on what you will do for your parent and stick to them. Don't cancel your vacation or leave work for the eighth time this week. If you are walking out the door and your father accuses you of neglecting him, . . . be clear and reassuring. '*I know it feels that way. It must be very hard living here alone. But I will be back on Tuesday, and you need to know that I am never going to abandon you.*'"[7]

Remember, in all relationships, that empathy goes a long way. Listening to your elderly loved one shows the love you have for him or her. You can acknowledge those feelings of anxiety or fear of abandonment without giving in to burdensome, unreasonable demands.

Mrs. Duncan no longer drives, but the siblings haven't been able to convince her to let them sell her car to spare the expense of auto insurance. The elderly woman says she likes looking out the window at her automobile in the parking lot and wants Daniel to drive it when he comes to look after her. Unfortunately, Mrs. Duncan's monthly expenses far exceed her Social Security income. Janet and her siblings hope her resources last to the end of her life and know they'll have to sell the car sometime soon.

An expert bridge player before the dementia onset, Mrs. Duncan can still play cards because her partners were never as good at bridge, so all are on an equal skill level now. She has a boyfriend who visits her most days in the late afternoon. Knowing her social competencies will decline as her cognitive impairments progress, Janet, Daniel, and Myra are grateful their mother still has a considerable quality of life. They take things one day at a time.

Problem behaviors and too few solutions can make *anyone's* best efforts at caregiving for their parent seem paltry, even when the situation hasn't quite yet become overwhelming. Janet, Daniel, and Myra consider themselves fortunate that their mother's financial resources have allowed them to care for her as they do now. When her savings are exhausted, they may find it more of a struggle, but they'll continue trying to do the best job of taking care of their mother that they know how to do.

HONORING OUR PARENTS

The stories I've shared show how hard—and how rewarding—it can be to care for our parents, even if they aren't able to express their gratitude. In virtually every culture across the globe, taking care of our parents in their old age is a core value widely shared. "Honor your father and mother" is one of Ten Commandments in the ancient scriptures of both Christians and Jews. Muslims, Hindus, Buddhists, Unitarians, and secular humanists share a similar sense of moral responsibility for providing caregiving to their elderly family members.

In the words of Mother Teresa, upon receiving the Nobel Peace Prize, "What can you do to promote world peace? Go home and love your family."[8] Echoing a similar set of values, Eleanor Roosevelt was quoted as saying, "Where after all, do universal human rights begin? In small places, close to home."[9]

In the Quran it is written, "Your Lord has commanded that you should worship none but Him, and show kindness to your parents. If either or both of them attain old age with you, say no word of contempt to them and do not rebuke them, but always speak gently to them and treat them with humility and tenderness and say, 'Lord, be merciful to them both, as they raised me up when I was little.'"[10]

Rabbi Shagra Simmons tells us, "We honor parents simply because they gave us the gift of life . . . By honoring those who brought us into existence, we learn not to take things for granted and develop an appreciation for the kindness of others."[11]

As I listen to caregivers like Lillian and Janet, more of Rabbi Simmons' advice on how to deal with the difficult parent comes to mind: "While honoring your parents is a tremendous mitzvah [commandment], you also need to be responsible for your own welfare. One is not required to endanger his emotional or physical health for a parent. Therefore, if a child cannot cope with the parent's behavior, he is permitted to keep his distance."[12]

Lillian lived by her Christian values and provided the oversight care for her father, even though he was a selfish man difficult to love. She also was kind to her father out of respect for her deceased mother and did the good job of taking care of him that her mother would have wanted. Lillian's siblings admired their sister's good heart and her ability to rise above their father's mistreatment of her (as a child and adult) to care for him in his old age.

Similarly, Janet and her siblings have arranged for the care of their mother, without causing her to feel that she is a burden or that they are looking after her only out of obligation. Janet, her caregiving brother, and their sister find ways to show kindness and love to their mother without being manipulated. Without guilt, they also take good care of their own health and make time for their spouses, grandchildren, and friends.

Whatever our religion or if we are not religious at all, whether caring for a parent or another loved one, a time will come when it is *our* turn to be on the receiving end. How can we hope to be regarded with respect by those who will look after *us* in our old age or frailty if we are not living by the Golden Rule? We treat others as we want to be treated because it's the right thing to do. In addition, there is truth to the old adage that "what goes around comes around."

MOST PEOPLE CAN'T AFFORD PAID HELP

If you are a caregiver, you are not alone. About one in every four adults in the United States provides unpaid care to an aging family member. Many of these family caregivers struggle to piece together the high-difficulty puzzle of providing elder care. Hiring someone to provide in-home care is affordable to only 10 to 20 percent of Americans, who lack government-sponsored home-helper systems like those in Denmark, Sweden, and Japan.[13]

If you're like most caregivers, you have to navigate the caregiving journey with limited financial resources. Handling one stressful situation or problem-solving crisis after another is enough to make anyone weary. According to Laura Berk in her internationally published book, *Development Through the Lifespan*, the burden tends to fall more on women than on men, showing itself in "role overload and high job absenteeism" and resulting in an "exhausting inability to concentrate, feelings of hostility, anxiety about aging, [and] high rates of depression."[14] Your own feelings about the challenges of caregiving are probably what led you to look for helpful tips and hopeful insights, like those I provide in this book.

The fact is that providing care for your impaired loved one has a learning curve as steep as the one many of us had as parents. Time and again over the years, just as we thought we had the "mom or dad thing" down, some baffling issue would arise that would cause us to worry, struggle with conflicting feelings, and doubt ourselves. Whether parenting our young children or "parenting" an elderly adult, we inevitably will make some poor decisions, simply because we are human beings. If we're not mindful, we will "trip over the rugs" of our mistakes made with the best of intentions—and a lack of knowledge. We can use all the help we can get from others who have had to learn things from trial and error as well as from medical professionals and other experts.

Researchers tell us that dementia advances more slowly when caregivers and care recipients share close, loving relationships and familiar, stimulating environments. What helps most to slow both functional and cognitive decline are "problem-solving coping [strategies that] lead to more effective caregiving and lower emotional stress in the caregiver."[15]

THE ABCS OF EFFECTIVE CAREGIVING INTERACTIONS

What is so difficult is adjusting to the constantly changing demands of caregiving. Just as you successfully master the art of handling one set of problem behaviors, your loved one's impairments increase to a new level. Your hard-won "skills may not always generalize to new caregiving challenges," explains Susan M. McCurry, a University of Washington research professor.

A much-in-demand expert in advising both geriatric professionals and family caregivers, McCurry offers a bounty of beneficial, practical guidance.[16] In a recent workshop, she gave a long list of common behaviors that caregivers find challenging: "crying and tearfulness, waking you and other family members at night, asking the same question over and over, getting dressed incorrectly or inappropriately, accusing people of stealing, trying to leave or leaving the house, getting lost inside or outside of the house, having temper outbursts, grabbing or clinging to you or other people, refusing to accept appropriate help with personal care, seeing or hearing things that aren't there, expressing feelings of hopelessness or loneliness, or making comments about feeling worthless or being a burden."[17]

McCurry goes on to describe the kinds of caregiving interactions most likely to be successful in addressing these problems: Caregivers should first focus on behaviors that threaten safety, interfere with care, or compromise the quality of life for either the giver or receiver of care. Next, look outward to community resources for adult day care programs that benefit the person with dementia while providing you with respite (a regular break, several times a week) to help prevent caregiver burnout. Look also to your own internal resources, McCurry advises: "Changing your response to behaviors can reduce their duration, severity, and probability of occurring in the future."[18]

In the words of Dr. J. Raymond DePaulo, until recently the chief of psychiatry at the Johns Hopkins University Medical Institutions, one of the most important lessons of caregiving is to "prevent the catastrophic reaction."[19] By keeping the cognitively impaired elder's environment as familiar and comfortable as possible, the communication respectful and caring, and by employing effective caregiver skills, troublesome behaviors often can be mitigated before they get out of hand.

It is still possible to have some kind of meaningful relationship with the precious human being whose neurocognitive disease is progressing. Glenn, a devoted husband, and Grace, who is suffering with a gradually worsening dementia, are featured in *Grace: The Alzheimer's Documentary.* Glenn involves Grace in activities that she has always enjoyed. He helps "cue" her to follow the familiar steps of dressing and feeding herself, slowing down his wife's loss of independence as much as possible. Recalling a scene from the documentary as we spoke, Dr. DePaulo quoted this loving husband: "If I can help her, I'll get more of Grace for longer."[20]

To help caregivers manage difficult behaviors, McCurry recommends that they follow an approach called "the ABCs of behavior change," developed by

Dr. Linda Teri at the University of Washington.[21] This approach guides the caregiver through three steps:

A—*Activator*: What happened before the behavior?

B—*Behavior*: What exactly was the person with dementia doing? Paint a verbal picture!

C—*Consequence*: What happened after the behavior?

Using this approach, caregivers work on one behavior at a time, choosing from one of the "4 Ws": "What was the person with dementia doing? Where did it happen? Who was there? When did it happen?" Caregivers are then instructed to identify what happened before the behavior occurred (activator), what happened after (consequence), and two or three ways the activator or consequence could be changed. In her workshop,[22] Dr. McCurry illustrated the A-B-C approach on a form developed by Dr. Teri and reproduced on the following page.

Elsewhere McCurry offers more practical steps for dealing with behavior changes. In *When a Family Member Has Dementia*, McCurry advises caregivers to DANCE, an acronym that spells out guidelines: "Don't argue. Accept realistic limitations. Nurture yourself. Creative problem-solving [through following] the ABCs of behavior change. Enjoy the moment."[23] In *Treating Dementia in Context: A Step-by-Step Guide*, she further offers the acronym POLITE, reminding caregivers to "watch nonverbal cues: be polite!" The types of caregiving interactions most likely to be successful in problem solving are "Patience, Organization, Laughter, Ignoring behaviors not harmful to self or others, Tone of voice, and Eye contact."[24]

Special kinds of abbreviations and acronyms can be lifesavers, such as HAZMAT for hazardous materials and FAST (warning you to act quickly to signs of a stroke): Face drooping, Arm weakness, or Speech difficulty—Time to call 911. *When you are stressed, an emotional lifesaver may be reminding yourself of the words DANCE and POLITE: focusing on their meanings may help steady you.*

INTENSIVE CAREGIVERS

If you are taking care of a loved one 21 hours a week or more, you have "the highest stress of all caregivers (a 4.4 rating out of 5)," according to a study recently reported in the *AARP Bulletin*.[25] In an article entitled, "When Caregiving

A-B-C Problem Solving Plan

Activator

What happens before? Mr. S. went into the bathroom then walked to the kitchen and walked outside. He told Mrs. S. when she ran after him that he was going to work.

Behavior

What is the person doing? Mr. S. leaves the house in the middle of the night.

Where does it happen? He exits out the kitchen door.

Who is there? Mr. & Mrs. S.

When does it happen? ~2 a.m., Tuesday night

Consequence

What happens after? Mrs. S. yelled, "You've been retired for 15 years!" and brought him back.

Get Active: Making Change Happen!

How could you possibly change the activators?

1. Hide Mr. S.'s robe and shoes when he first goes to bed.

2. Hang curtain in hallway so Mr. S. doesn't see the door.

3. Move deadbolt on door so it's harder for Mr. S. to figure out how to open it.

How might you change the consequences?

1. Get up when Mr. S. goes to the bathroom and invite him nicely to come back to bed as soon as he finishes.

2. Don't try to explain that he is retired so he doesn't need to work. Don't yell or argue!!!

Circle your best ideas to try this week!!!

Linda Teri, *Managing and Understanding Behavior Problems in Alzheimer's Disease and Related Disorders* (training program with videotapes and written manual) (Seattle: University of Washington, 1990). Reproduced with permission of Dr. Linda Teri.

Is Round the Clock," the story is told of Estelle Sandler, 68, "who is at the intensive end of the caregiving spectrum, spending most of the day assisting her partner, Angie DiPrinzio, who is working to overcome the effects of a stroke."[26]

DiPrinzio was a personal trainer and active athlete when complications of having a supposedly routine root canal led to an infection, a blood clot, and stroke. Although "the couple's life has been uprooted since 2008 . . . Sandler, a retired teacher, has been helping DiPrinzio regain her balance, as well as relearn tasks as simple as folding laundry and turning on the tap water."[27]

What helps Sandler mitigate such a high level of stress is cherishing their loving relationship, seeing how hard DiPrinzio works to continue her recovery at home and at a stroke recovery center, and having four hours to herself every weekday while her spouse takes advantage of the stroke rehabilitation facility. Sandler's spirits are also uplifted by having discovered strengths within herself, strengths well beyond what she could have imagined before nearly losing her life partner.[28]

TAKE ADVANTAGE OF THE MANY AVAILABLE RESOURCES

Paula Spencer Scott, an author with four close family members who have had dementia, offers "soul saving wisdom for caregivers" in her 2014 book, *Surviving Alzheimer's*. And in the November 2015 *AARP Bulletin* article, "Places That Lend a Hand," Scott names three of the best places to start reducing your caregiver stress by matching the available resources in your community with your particular needs:

1. To find "Your local Area Agency on Aging . . . go to n4a.org." Programs are available at these government-funded agencies, Scott continues, offering "respite care, support groups, education and training and emergency assistance."
2. For information on "adult day programs, financial and legal assistance, housing options, in-home services and more," she recommends calling 800-677-1116 or going to eldercare.gov/eldercare.net/public/index.aspx.
3. Additionally, to find a state-by-state listing of services and programs for family caregivers, the Family Caregiver Alliance is a godsend: "Go online to caregiver.org/family-care-navigator."[29]

The Alzheimer's Association is a nonprofit organization with a national website offering information on every imaginable issue of concern related to

"Alzheimer's disease and dementia symptoms, diagnosis, stages, treatment, care, and support services." You will find at www.alz.org a toll-free Helpline with a number you can call 24/7. Anytime—day or night—you can call to talk with someone at 1-800-272-3900. The website tells how to access an amazing wealth of available resources around the country, and it provides invaluable information and an online library through which you can find an up-to-date supply of educational materials. Also available is detailed information about agencies that provide respite services, including day care programs and volunteer or paid caregivers who come into the home to care for an impaired person to give family caregivers relief for hours or days at a time, and videos that entertain and comfort patients with dementia.

VIDEO RESOURCES FOR CAREGIVERS

You can learn about "respite videos" by watching an excellent six-minute YouTube film entitled, "Alzheimer's Respite Video—Mom Watching for the Very First Time." The Alzheimer's Association at https://www.alz.org/library has a valuable supply of other videos that are meant to engage, entertain, and stimulate the person with dementia. Meaningfully occupying your loved one for a short time can provide you with an opportunity to do cleaning jobs around the house, read a magazine, or otherwise have a break from the often intense, nonstop stress of caregiving. Other videos include songs likely to be familiar to your loved one and may encourage dialogue between the person speaking or singing in the video and your impaired elder.

Respite videos have been shown in studies to be more effective in keeping the attention of the person with dementia than watching *Lawrence Welk*, although "champagne music" and dancing programs are far better for the elderly person than watching regular TV. Some older folks will briefly be entertained by videos of slow-moving and very basic 1950s or 1960s TV programs like *I Love Lucy*, *Father Knows Best*, and *Hogan's Heroes*, or shows for young children such as *Mr. Rogers' Neighborhood*, *Sesame Street*, or *The Roy Rogers and Dale Evans Show*. Similarly, only recordings of music that are known to be calming and remain pleasing to the impaired elder should be played.

Information is available through the same https://www.alz.org/library website for obtaining caregiver resources that are free, such as *La Familia Latina y Problemas de la Memoria: La Enfermedad de Alzheimer*. You can purchase (for about $30) *Facing Alzheimer's: An African American Perspective*. For professionals, at the cost of approximately $150, is the (Dr. Peter V.) *Rabins Response to the Challenging Behaviors of Alzheimer's Disease*, produced by Video Press, the University of Maryland School of Medicine. Many other available videos provide activities including favorite sing-along songs and resources for caregivers, plus educational videos for both laypeople and professionals.

A creative person, not too burdened, with the energy and time, can make meaningful and personalized videos. Gerontology professors Dale A. Lund and colleagues, in "Video Respite: An Innovative Resource for Family, Professional Caregivers, and Persons with Dementia," say homemade videos can be effective if the content is positive, slow paced, focuses on long-term memories familiar to the person with dementia, features only one person talking on screen, and encourages interaction from the elder with dementia.[30]

Having a household membership in AARP so that you can receive their monthly *Bulletin* and semimonthly AARP *The Magazine* is another way to stay abreast of available resources and get helpful advice. You will find a regularly replenishing supply of informative articles and uplifting personal stories. The *Bulletin*'s "Random Acts of Kindness for Caregivers," for example, sparked in my mind some of the ideas that follow.

WHAT TO SAY WHEN OTHERS OFFER TO HELP OR WOULD HELP IF YOU ASKED

Many of us aren't very good at letting others know when the stress we're feeling and the problems we're constantly endeavoring to solve are making us tread water. If there was ever a time and place for reaching out for all the support you can get, it's when you have that heavily fatigued caregiver feeling of fighting not to drown.

Perhaps you know another caregiver who would be willing to trade off watching both of the people each of you help so you can each have regular free time to spend as you want? Is there a teenage or adult grandchild who would be glad to do some "grandma sitting" or earn some spending money by helping out with chores at your house or running errands? Might you ask one of the volunteers delivering Meals on Wheels to provide you with respite time a few hours each week for some kind of payment?

When others ask how they can help or would be glad to help if you asked, you can choose from the ideas below or come up with your own specific requests. Especially if your caregiving is virtually round the clock, you need to *allow* a friend, family member, neighbor, or someone from your community organization, church, or synagogue to help out. Just say, "Yes, thanks! I would really appreciate your helping me by . . .

- picking up a prescription [or a couple days' worth of groceries, some dog food, birdseed, items at the dry cleaners or something at the post office];
- cooking a hot meal and bringing it over at dinnertime to drop off or to stay and share;
- coming over to help decorate the house for the holidays [or to rake leaves, clean gutters, shovel snow, or cut the grass];
- gifting a prepaid card to a spa for a massage, manicure, or pedicure;
- keeping company with the elderly loved one for several hours on a certain day *every week* to make possible an exercise or yoga class [book club, weekly swim, tennis game or gym workout, card game, or movie or dinner date with a friend];
- coming over to 'elder sit' on special occasions, enabling attendance at a religious service or concert, grandchild's birthday party, or sporting event;
- lending an ear on the phone or going out to lunch together, with the opportunity to ventilate some annoyances, worries, or problems that need to be figured out;
- getting together for lunch or doing something that sounds fun, just to enjoy having a break from caregiving and talking about *anything else*."[31]

JUST DON'T WAIT UNTIL YOU'RE BURNED OUT

"Once a rewarding, enjoyable life has been lost," writes psychologist Laura Berk, "it is difficult to restore. Furthermore, frequent, regular respite is far more helpful than infrequent, irregular use. Caregivers who end up spending respite hours doing housework, shopping, or working usually remain dissatisfied. Those who engage in activities they had wanted and planned to do gain in psychological well-being."[32]

Organizations like AARP, the National Alliance for Caregiving, your local

Department of Aging, and community groups can help you and your family find free resources that are available to assist you through difficult times. You probably won't be surprised to learn that women and men cope differently. In research on coping strategies that was done for AARP in 2013, Linda Barrett found that "female caregivers are hungry for solitary activities, time to read a good book, go for a walk or to the gym," while "male caregivers would choose spending uninterrupted time with a spouse, going to a movie or sporting event or other recreational activity." Among the caregivers Barrett studied, women were more likely than men to talk with others (45 percent vs. 29 percent) and to pray or meditate (59 percent vs. 44 percent), both of which are positive coping strategies. On the negative side, however, the females were more likely than their male counterparts to smoke (16 percent vs. 9 percent), more likely to put off making tough decisions (37 percent vs. 28 percent), and less likely to use exercise as a way of coping (14 percent vs. 21 percent).[33]

"You aren't fit to take care of other people if you're not wise enough to take care of yourself!" These words provided one of the first lessons my supervisors taught me when I began to look after patients as a student in a hospital chaplaincy course at Duke University Medical Center. The advice was valuable later when I was a psychology intern working with psychiatric inpatients at Johns Hopkins. Whether we are in a professional helping role or assuming the responsibilities of a family caregiver, the importance of not trying to be the steel-driving man who worked himself to death is a lesson worth remembering and heeding.

Getting yourself into a routine of daily exercise is probably the best thing you can do to stay well and feel stronger as a caregiver. Countless well-designed scientific studies have robustly demonstrated that exercise reduces the risk of depression, illness, and injuries.

Regular exercise gives us the best chance we have to help ourselves live longer, happier lives. There is a dark humor in a cartoon by Glasbergen that made me smile: A doctor in a white coat is speaking to an unfit middle-aged guy standing in his underwear in the examining room. Says the doctor, "What fits your busy schedule better, exercising one hour a day or being dead 24 hours a day?"[34]

However slowly paced our daily walk or walks, we will move faster than any couch potato is likely to race. It doesn't matter so much how fast we move or how far we walk, we can gradually increase the time, distance, and speed.[35] It's a life-giving activity.

As a caregiver, in order for *you* to sustain a balanced life that protects and promotes good physical and mental health, getting respite time to engage in enjoyable activities—*at least twice a week for several hours*—is essential.[36]

Caregiving is hard work. There's no other way to surmount the challenges of elder care: to find the best life within reach, you have to take good care of yourself.

Comforting Insights and Myth-Busting Knowledge

Stress is a sign of a meaningful life. Let's start looking at it that way.
—Sanjay Gupta, MD

At times it's hard for us to grasp the idea that feeling dispirited or burdened is not simply the result of circumstances beyond our control. Certain hardships and sorrows in our lives can feel like speeding trucks heading our way, threatening to smash us flat like miniature cars turned into pieces of metal.

It isn't easy to think of stress as something manageable, let alone beneficial, especially when you're a caregiver weary from nights of being unable to fall asleep or stay asleep. Worries come constantly to mind, problems to solve, and sad feelings you try not to think about.

There is valuable knowledge and there are ways of thinking, however, that can help you turn some quite miserable things into events that will give your life renewed meaning. A key concept in psychology is the perspective that our feelings come from our thoughts and expectations; therefore, if we change how we think about an ordeal we're trying to cope with, we can change how we feel. Worth pondering are these words: *as you expect to experience an experience, so you will experience that experience.* Put another way, by author Shawn Achor, "90 percent of your long-term happiness depends on the way you process the world in which you find yourself."[1]

MYTH #1

It Doesn't Matter What I Do, They Won't Remember It Anyway

My friend Carrie, just back from Chicago after spending a good-quality long weekend with her elderly parents, phones them when her plane lands in Baltimore. It doesn't matter if you are 18, 28, or 58 (Carrie's age), parents like to know that you're back home safely. You didn't die. The airplane didn't crash.

Carrie's dad answers the phone. "Hi, Carrie," he says. "When are you going to come see us?"

"Sometimes," Carrie told me, "I say, 'Dad, I was just there.' Many times, it's not worth correcting. It doesn't matter. I just ask Dad what he had for lunch. He turns to my mother and I can hear him speaking to her. 'What did I have for lunch?' Then Dad says, 'It was a tuna fish sandwich and it was good.'"

Why is it that Carrie *often* makes such long trips? Why does a late afternoon rarely pass without a phone conversation shared with each of her parents, as she drives to a meeting or travels home from work? *Why? Because Carrie loves her parents and is a kind-hearted daughter.* In addition to all the ways that she and her spouse help her parents financially, does all the time Carrie spends trying to give her folks emotional support really count for anything? *Yes, even though her mother tearfully complains a great deal and seems always to need more time than Carrie can give, her many visits uplift the spirits of* both *parents.*

She is the very busy chief financial officer managing a $270 million budget for an academic institution. Because times are economically difficult for colleges and universities nationwide, Carrie is constantly up late. She manages a large staff, works hard to find new ways to save money, and builds budgets that earn the support of the government officials and agencies that fund higher education. She has a wife, an extended family, and her own health issues (cancer in remission) to look after, too. Most especially, why does Carrie *always* ask to talk to her dad—even though he will have forgotten their phone conversation only minutes after they've said good-bye? With his advanced Alzheimer's disease, does her dad even "get it" that he is cared about? *Of course he does!*

As every caregiver of an elderly person knows, there are good times and bad. Often periods of near-normal functioning and lucidity are interspersed with periods of great impairment or distress. Until profound disability sets in or the end nears, elders with physical or cognitive problems or both are unpredictably better or worse from one day or hour to the next.

Fortunately for both of them, Carrie's dad had a lucid moment when he was able to initiate a call to his daughter to say that he loved her—less than 24 hours before he died. Part of her dad was still "there" right up to his last moments of breath. So it is with others, even those with some form of dementia more advanced than his: *love given and kindness expressed endure, make a lasting impact, whether or not the person on the receiving end can express gratitude or even mumble an acknowledgement.*

False Assumptions

Assuming that your loved one is so impaired that there is scarcely any quality of life left in his or her future is the first myth to replace. I say this because there is some good news about the aging process. Even if your loved one has progressively severe brain damage, there is reason for hope. In his excellent book, *I'm Still Here: A New Philosophy of Alzheimer's Care*, John Zeisel writes that, despite the fact that someone with Alzheimer's may have lost 10 or 20 or 30 *billion* brain cells, 90 or 80 or 70 *billion* brain cells remain active. As he explains, "Alzheimer's disease damages the brain, but a lot of the brain still functions. Those cells hold hope! . . . The good news is that a great deal is going on in there even as our brains get plaques, tangles, cavities, folds, and fissures."[2]

Zeisel emphasizes that hardwired abilities exist, "sometimes called instincts or natural feelings," that make it possible for "people living with Alzheimer's to communicate with us and we with them." He mentions "facial expressions, responses to the touch of another, singing, and landmarks of way-finding—all abilities that last our entire lives." Zeisel goes on to explain that "the need for contact with the natural environment and the feelings we have about nature and being outdoors are hardwired," too. "Sunshine, flowers, shade, moonlight, and trees are all so much a part of our basic nature that no one has to be taught to respond appropriately to such stimuli."[3]

Creating supportive environments (including familiar furniture, wall hangings, photos, and walkways that cue the brain for way-finding but keep a person safe) and improving caregiver communication skills are ways to still share satisfying experiences with your loved one. *There is a quality of life still possible for both of you.*

Caring and Acts of Kindness Are Deeply Experienced— but Not "Felt Meanings"

When I first visited my much-beloved grandmother in an Arizona nursing home, I saw that Granny's memory was failing, but she still recognized me as her granddaughter. When I handed her a bound copy of my recently completed doctoral dissertation, she held it in her hands and looked through it for what seemed a long time, acknowledged the meaning of it, and beamed with pride. Even 37 years later, I have a vivid picture of her and deeply cherish that satisfied look on Granny's face. More than anyone else in my life, this dear woman— who was born in 1891 and had an eighth-grade education—was unfaltering in her encouragement as I pursued my educational goals and dreams. Granny had long been a steadying influence when I struggled financially and battled self-doubt. My given middle name is Marie, making me Granny's namesake. After I shared my dissertation with her, she always wrote "Dr. Ann Marie" on the envelopes that enclosed her loving letters. Occasionally Granny similarly addressed and enclosed a bank check written out for "one dollar," with the word "treat" added in ink on the subject line. As a young college teacher, I loved taking those checks to the payroll window and cashing them!

A year or so after my first visit, when I traveled from Maryland across the country to visit her in the nursing home, my eyes filled with tears as I saw "how far gone" she was. While my mother pushed Granny's wheelchair and I stepped back to follow them into the garden area, Granny said, "Is she crying?" My mother, not knowing what else to say, replied that I was not.

In hindsight, a better response would have been for my mother to say, "Yes. Ann Marie is crying because she's your granddaughter and she's so glad to see you. She loves you very much." Regardless, I realize now that Granny was able to enjoy the familiarity of our faces even if she hadn't recognized exactly who we were. And (once an awesome flower grower and charter member of her local garden club), Granny was still able to cherish the sunshine and enjoy being wheeled around through a maze of multicolored flowerbeds.

One of those hard-wired abilities—even in advanced Alzheimer's disease— is the recognition of human facial expressions that bespeak sadness, anger, disgust or contempt, fear and pleasure.[4] Psychologist Rodolfo ("Rudy") Zea shared his perspectives with me in a personal conversation not long ago. Assisted living and nursing home residents, explained Dr. Zea, when able to tell us what they feel, express three concerns: (1) their family members don't visit enough; (2) they would like to see family members *happier* when they do visit;

and (3) it is a matter of politeness and respect to "be of good cheer," and *not* to show them pity![5]

Just as both positive and negative emotions are picked up by an infant or child and are mirrored in return, so too does an elderly loved one in our care recognize the emotions that our facial expressions reflect. Even if they don't understand what is being "said" nonverbally, their mood can pick up the energy conveyed. For this reason, troublesome feelings need to be ventilated to a friend, pastoral counselor, or psychologist or written in a private journal. Then, when we're in the presence of our loved one, our faces and our words can better offer genuine expressions of calmness, caring, and pleasure.

In my late 30s, I returned to Baltimore. Grieving what I'd seen in Arizona as my grandmother's miserable condition, I went to a therapist who was an older woman physician and mentor to me in those days. Thankfully, the psychiatrist's insights into Granny's mental and emotional capacities gave me a new and comforting perspective: "Your grandmother no longer has *felt meanings*," Dr. Joffe explained. "*You* feel sorry for her but she doesn't have the ability to feel sorry for *herself*."

I learned then that we must be capable of *interpreting* events and applying such insight to our own circumstances, in order to experience mourning. Interpretation is a complex mental ability perhaps blessedly taken from a person in my Granny's situation. Unlike in early Alzheimer's, when people inevitably are frustrated and greatly saddened by their worsening cognitive losses, those with advanced dementia are unable to hold such complex perspectives in their mind long enough to give them *sustained* feelings. The ability to interpret events and apply those meanings to ourselves and our loved ones is how we experience deeply felt emotions like the sorrow I felt for my Granny. Understanding that *she* no longer had the capacity for such insight and ruminating thoughts made me glad for her and less sad on her behalf. The grief work that needed to be done was all mine.

But Granny *could* still experience and respond to the familiarity of our faces and be calmed by the playing or singing of familiar hymns. She could still absorb nature's beauty in the garden areas surrounding the nursing home. Granny's spirit also seemed soothed when one of us stood gently combing her hair or sat tenderly stroking her hand. A cynic observing this might say, "Oh, but it's all for naught! Two minutes after you leave, she won't even know you came all the way across the country to visit her." (This is, of course, a common but not carefully considered excuse many family members give themselves for staying away entirely.)

From Birth to the Grave: Every Act of Caring *Is* Received

Yes, Granny would forget that we had been there as soon as we left her sight, and she forgot that we were her daughter and granddaughter even while we were all still sitting together in the afternoon sun. However, now that I've raised my own children, I see my previously depressing, negative way of looking at things quite differently. The love we give our very young children, I realize, is very much like the love we give our very old parents. Reciprocity and our child or parent being aware of "getting it" aren't the point.

My grown daughters probably don't realize how much I loved each of them and prayed for their health and for the well-being of their little hearts long before they were born. In their early 30s now, they mostly don't remember the air travel, limo rides, and countless hotel stays I warmly recall our sharing when they were infants and little girls. We played games, read stories, enjoyed "room service," and visited amusement parks thanks to my publishers letting me take my family along everywhere on business trips. Of course, my adult daughters also don't remember hundreds of loving times shared in rocking chairs, on neighborhood walks, playgrounds, sandy beaches, and long car rides as babies and toddlers. Still, those experiences are an integral part of my daughters' very essence as persons and *within their hearts forever*—and so are all of the loving times we share with our impaired elderly loved ones, whether they "remember" them or not.

No one remembers the nurturance they received in their parents' arms from birth to the age of three, but every major study in psychology verifies that without that nurturance, all of us would literally have died. Just as we pat the back, massage the little head, sing and talk to a tiny baby who can't tell us that he or she is taking it all in, so we continue to speak loving words and hold the hand of a loved one in a coma or in hospice care. We continue to relate actively to our impaired elderly loved one because that care *is* being received—whether acknowledged or not—and *does* provide nourishment.

This reality can comfort you and give meaning to every act of kindness you offer. Warm experiences in our loved ones' lives do not have to be "remembered" to become an ongoing part of their physical, emotional, and spiritual memory.

Loving care and a familiar, more stimulating environment are among the reasons why the functional decline of dementia has been shown to advance more slowly in closer caregiver-patient relationships. For spouses caring for a loved one with Alzheimer's disease and other loving caregivers, what helps most to slow the progression of both physical disabilities and cognitive decline are problem-solving strategies that lead to more effective caregiving. In addition, studies show that lowering *your* emotional stress as a caregiver can greatly improve your loved one's quality of life.[6]

MYTH #2

In Old Age, We Become Like Children Again

I'm sure *I* don't want to be thought of or treated like a child when I'm old or become physically or mentally disabled. Do *you*? Doesn't just the idea of it feel like a disgraceful, degrading way for our family caregivers to think of us, after all our years of loving and providing for them? After contributing to our communities and giving our hearts and the fruits of our labor to our children, grandchildren, other relatives, and friends — how sad and how insulting if our fate is to be categorized and marginalized in our sundown years!

As a psychology intern in the 1970s, I learned many "forever lessons" from a wonderful physician teacher at the Johns Hopkins University Medical Institutions. Dr. Phillip Slavney taught me that there is always an adult person to be known, valued, and respected in every patient. Whether the person is sick, frail, or severely mentally ill, we fail the people we care for as professionals if we don't look for our patients' strengths and affirm them. There is a lesson here for family members as well.

"Let's not batter our loved ones to death with our own expectations," said Dr. Rodolfo Zea, when I interviewed this humanist and expert in gerontology. "When the needs of elderly people are not understood, they have reason to be depressed and angry," he continued. "The ultimate gift is to set a standard for growing old with dignity and grace, by realizing that we all want respect. We all want to be understood. What life is all about is being tolerant, being kind, and learning forgiveness." For more than a decade as the psychologist at a Baltimore residential community and multilevel care facility for seniors, Dr. Zea kept emphasizing that "I got as much benefit therapeutically from my interaction with these residents as they got from me. When families can just respect their elders, *they* also may receive more than they give."

Over the years, as her mother's Alzheimer's disease progressed, my friend Marian realized that her beloved mother required (and, together with her brother and father, saw to it that she received) full-time nursing care. Although

Mrs. Misemer could still dress herself every day until she suffered the stroke that led to her death, the elderly woman's ability to reason and to remember life-altering events, like her brother's death, and daily tasks, such as eating and taking her medications, were quite severely impaired. Fortunately for both of them, Marian's ways of responding to her mother never wavered in being loving and respectful. "I'd never want to argue that my mother wasn't a person until the moment she died," Marian told me.

"It's so important to know that [people with dementia] aren't infants, they're not their disease. They are people with needs and you can communicate with them," explains Lisa Snyder. A social worker, Snyder cautions family members to take care not to communicate negativity through body language that signals stress or irritation.[7] It is also crucial, writes journalist Janice Lynch Schuster in the *Washington Post*, to be a good listener, to reflect back the emotions or concerns you hear being expressed (even if she or he seems not to be making sense). Then try to change the subject to say how much you love each other or reminisce about experiences you've shared.[8]

"Just because you have dementia," Dr. Zea explained, "that doesn't mean you don't recall some things that happened a long time ago; or that you might not appreciate poetry, or music, or that you are not sensitive. There is always something important to these residents regardless of whether it is important to others. The more you realize that your loved one will never be completely gone, even when it seems that way, they will always leave you with some notion of themselves. In this light, they are the therapists."

In the story of Marlene and her mother that follows, Dr. Zea's comforting insights are driven home: "We must see with our minds and hearts—not just with our eyes—in order to understand how *they* [our impaired elderly loved ones] *are the therapists.*"

MYTH #3

There's Nothing They Can Do for *Me* Anymore; I Do All the Giving

Marlene's mother is 79. Her doctor told the family that Mrs. Williams had "early-onset Alzheimer's disease" when she was 58 or 59 in 1995, but that was almost surely a misdiagnosis. It seems impossible to me that could have been a correct diagnosis since that kind of early-onset dementia strikes young and typically progresses rapidly, and Mrs. Williams lived self-sufficiently for many years after that. After her husband died in 1997, she continued to drive and thrive. It was eight long years after the diagnosis before Mrs. Williams went to Virginia to visit another daughter and called Marlene to say, "I can't remember where I live!"

By 2006, "Mom's condition got so bad," Marlene told me, "that she could no longer be left alone. She still lives in her own house with my sister, sister's daughter, and Mom's seven-year-old great-granddaughter—four generations." Mrs. Williams is severely cognitively impaired, but she is a hardy woman, spiritually and physically strong. "My mom endured a lot," Marlene explained. "My mother was one of 10 children. She grew up in South Carolina and picked cotton as a child. Her father (my grandfather) was a stern man. He was a farmer, a sharecropper. He was descended from a man who was a slave, fathered by his slave master." Fortunately, Mrs. Williams grew up to live a happy life with a good husband (Marlene describes him as an "awesome dad"), a man employed all his working years with Bethlehem Steel in its heyday, enabling Mrs. Williams to be a stay-at-home mom for their five children. Their church and faith were and are at the center of the extended family's life, and over the years many ministers and deacons are counted among them.

Marlene is 50 years old, the mother of five and grandmother of three. She and her 10-year-old daughter live in their home, just a short distance from Mrs. Williams' house. Also living with Marlene is her grown daughter and the daughter's daughter, who is seven. While interviewing her, I am thinking that this is the textbook African American extended family—sharing in remarkable ways the load of providing caregiving for their elderly loved one. "My aunt took care of my grandmother until she died," Marlene tells me. "For both cultural and religious reasons, I could never put my mother in a nursing home." Marlene shoulders much of the caregiving, helped out by her four adult children, sister, brothers, and their children.

Some of life's deepest truths, I realize, are experienced in unexpected circumstances and are almost impossible to put into words. Marlene's humility and the deep meaning she has found in caring so lovingly for her mother have touched my heart. "When your parents have you, they never see taking care of *you* as a burden or problem," she says. It is a perspective that Marlene imagines would be obvious to everyone: "Mom took care of me. So taking care of *her* isn't a burden to me. She's just my mom."

Five days a week she prepares breakfast and lunch for her mother, dropping these meals at her mother's house on Tuesdays and Thursdays, on her way to school. While her sister is at work on those days, Marlene's niece is her mother's caregiver. On Monday, Wednesday, and Friday, Marlene stays at her mother's house or takes her mom to her own home or on errands and other trips in the car. I marvel at how she does it all and remains seemingly so young. She is a gentle soul with many obligations, trying to do a good job of caring for the four generations of family that she loves. Nonetheless, she is full of optimism. In the college classroom, where Marlene is the age of most of my students' parents, she is a bright and thoughtful person, with insights to share, and always eager to learn.

"This Has to Be a Life Lesson for Me"

"When I call her Mom, she always answers. Most days she knows I'm Marlene. But when I go to her every Monday through Friday, I don't know where she's going to be. I'm either going to join her in her happiness or try to bring her back to a more familiar place."

Continuing, Marlene explains, "Sometimes she's not the mother I know. She is a stranger walking around with clothes in her hands. It's like I'm loving the stranger, the person I don't know. My mother says, 'Somebody took my baby! I have to leave now!' She says she's waiting for *her* mother to come get her."

Marlene goes on to say that it's unconditional love that she feels at such times. "I don't know this person—but I know my mother is in there, and I have to try to reach that person. I've learned not to go against her. If she says something that is combative, I either agree with her or try to shift the conversation to something else. I will turn on some gospel music and start singing along. Lots of times, Mom will join in singing, too."

Having studied resilience and knowing that what resilient people do is learn something of benefit to themselves and others from the hardships they face, I'm struck by what Marlene tells me next: *"It's not just her illness,"* she says. *"This has to be a life lesson. God puts me in a certain place at a certain time. There's something in it for me."*

Always having been close as mother and daughter "makes it super easy for me to sacrifice for her," Marlene goes on. "It makes me more determined to survive the stress and pray much harder to have the energy needed. I have to give her back what she has given so unselfishly to me."

In recent weeks, her mother's condition has been getting worse. "She was always so nice, humble, and loving. She was never violent, but as her brain disease worsens, she has periods of agitation and lashing out," Marlene tells me.

The stress can feel unbearable. "So much has happened," Marlene goes on, "that I can't take it all in, or I'll be in tears and won't be able to function." How Marlene copes with it is "just to see my [caregiving] as work. This is something I have to do. It's part of my daily routine."

Marlene shares with me that she "definitely would feel the grief" if she let herself. "But you have to pick and choose what days and when you talk about watching a part of her dying every day. If you deal with the whole thing, it's too much."

Very frequently, Marlene calls Virginia to talk with her sister. "We talk almost every night, but we don't discuss my mother before bedtime. That's because if we don't get our sleep, we wouldn't want to face the next day."

Marlene says that although she has periods of feeling a deep sorrow and times of mourning what her mother has lost, she sees "a glimpse of who my mother used to be and still is. I see her moving her lips and praying, with a tear running down her cheek. I hear her say, 'Thank you, Jesus.' And I know that *she's still there.*"

"A Totally Different Way of Loving"

I ask Marlene if she is finding tremendous meaning in giving back to her mother. "Absolutely! It has taught me," she replies, "a totally different way of loving."

Her mother "loves to get out of the house and doesn't get combative," when Marlene takes her for a drive in the car or to the mall to walk. "She has a bad knee, so we walk slowly. She holds my arm, and enjoys seeing pretty things in the store windows."

About one thing Marlene is certain. "I'm going to treat Mom with the respect and dignity she deserves. I respect every part of her. I still shop for her and dress her like always, like she would do if she could do for herself."

Marlene explains that physically her mother is fine, but "mentally she struggles to have a complete thought. Her sentences are most times scrambled. She can't put together a sentence. If she engaged in a conversation, she would be trying to express something, but it would have nothing to do with the conversation you're having." For example, "If you said, 'Mom, how are you feeling?' She would reply, 'I didn't have anything to do with it. It was fine the last time I looked.'"

Coping with Costs

Solemnly, Marlene continued, "I'd be lying to you if I said there weren't days that you just want it to all go away—but never at the cost of losing her. I could never put my mother in a nursing home, but we're going to have to find some additional help."

Marlene was raised in a middle-class family in Baltimore City, "in a community that consisted mostly of two-parent homes," she explains. "My parents lived the American dream, and they raised us to believe you can have whatever you work for. Dad made sure that my mom would be fine financially—and she would have been, if she hadn't had Alzheimer's. When he died, the house and car were paid for. My parents had savings. But with a sickness like this, you have to have an enormous amount of money, and then you don't know how long your loved one is going to live."

One of the medicines Marlene's mother needed was "$500 for a bottle of 30 pills—just a month's supply of Aricept—but we paid it because we wanted to give her any help that could slow down the disease. Finally, something changed with the pharmacy, and now the insurance pays it. This illness is like, whew! I'm amazed that anyone can afford to pay for health care for a family member."

As if to put into bold print what I have not shared with her but have learned from studies that examine why African American families so rarely access support from government and community agencies, Marlene relates her own experiences. "My parents were prideful people. They always took care of themselves. So for me to seek help from a government agency just doesn't feel right."

But help *is* needed, even with an extended family of caregivers doing their share. Marlene closed her business (a beauty salon) to take care of her mother and to go back to school. "I was going to apply to a Baltimore City program that pays a family member to take care of an elderly person—until I learned there is a waiting list with 25,000 people already on it!" She carefully manages her family's finances and drives a sometimes-unreliable 12-year-old car so that she can continue her own education and send her daughter to a parochial elementary school.

Marlene also looked into a program that could provide her mother with day care, "but the cost was going to be hundreds of dollars every week—just for a few hours a day!" There ought to be a way in America, we agreed, as millions of baby boomers age, for countless families to find affordable help to care for their frail elderly loved ones.

"Even though I still work full time," I told Marlene, "I'm old enough to receive a monthly Social Security check, and I don't feel ashamed, because there's no stigma attached to receiving Social Security."

"Yes," Marlene replied, "there ought to be a *dignified* program—something like Social Security—for the government to assist families like ours."

One government-funded program she investigated, Marlene continued, "would provide a mere $200 a *year* for adult diapers, but they asked so many invasive personal questions, it was degrading. It was like begging to prove to an agency that my 79-year-old mother needs Depends!" Furthermore, "everything is too expensive or a dead end street with a long waiting list," Marlene lamented. "There are just not enough places to help Alzheimer's families. You have to have someone who is compassionate. If I try again to find help from some support groups, I fear I might be let down. If they let me down, I would really feel hopeless."

Determined to give her mother the best care possible under difficult circumstances Marlene keeps reminding herself that "a part of my mom is still there. On her birthday, Christmas, and Mother's Day, we always shower her with gifts. People say, 'Why bother?' Well, we're going to treat my mother just as if she will remember every bit of it!"

There are many terribly painful, hard times, Marlene acknowledges. "Some days, she just grabs my face or hand and says, 'Don't leave me!' She says, 'I can't think. It just won't come out!' It's so important to keep my mother a part of our lives. I rub her head. I touch her hands. I let her plant flowers and put her hands in the dirt, like she used to do as a farm girl." If Marlene asks one of her church friends or the Alzheimer's organization (alz.org) for help—to have even a few hours a week of respite—she could find some relief from the caregiving stress she so gladly carries.

Affirming her mother's worth, Marlene reemphasizes the stance she takes: "Even though Mom's words can still be scrambled, *she's still in there*. I see her. There are moments when parts of her peek out." An example of this concerns a longstanding joke in the family. "All my life," Marlene explained, "the card I played to get my way, as the youngest child, was to say that my oldest sister was Mom's favorite, and that I was the 'oops!' baby. Then Mom always said, 'No. No. That's not true. I treated you all the same. You're just different people. I love you all the same.' Well, recently, I said to my sister, Tanya, jokingly, not even thinking Mom was listening or would understand, 'Well, *you* were always

Mom's favorite.'" To Marlene's surprise, her mom then said, in words plain as day, "That's not true! I loved you all the same."

"God's Lesson"

"I'm just like anyone else," Marlene told me, sharing her honest yearnings. "I have ambition. I want to have a nice car, travel, and have nice things. Maybe what God wants me to learn is that it's not that I can't have those things. It's that I'm looking for one type of success, while there's something else greater that has nothing to do with material things."

Noting that she likes the curtains closed in her own home but that her mother likes them open, Marlene tells me that in the morning, at her own house or Marlene's place, her mom pulls back the curtains and says, "Oh, what a beautiful day!" Or when she can't find words, she just opens the window and says, "Ahhhh . . ."

With admiration, Marlene says, "When I see how she struggles but still appreciates sunshine and fresh air, I feel humbled. I definitely have learned to do less complaining, because I see my mother recognizing the beauty in just waking up. She doesn't have plans. She's not like you and I, but she can appreciate the day. That's amazing! Maybe my mission is to find a sense of peace with life and be thankful with just waking up."

MYTH #4

A Little Good Doesn't Matter

It is easy to feel insignificant, writes Father Joe Breighner, in a small book with a curious title, *For the Love of Stray Cats*. "In the grand scheme of things," we may ask ourselves, "what am I doing that really matters?" Comparing the pope's impact on the lives of millions of people to his own feeding and petting of two stray cats, this humble priest ponders how easily "we discount our individual acts of kindness . . . [and] discount ourselves."[9]

Whether you are a spiritually minded person or secular in how you ponder the meaning of your life, I think you may agree with Father Breighner when he says, "She got it right," and quotes Mother Theresa: "Most of us are not called to do great things. Most of us are called to do small things with great love."

"Put simply, no good is wasted," continues the man who preaches "lessons cats can teach us about living, loving, leaving, and letting go." He emphasizes that "the father changing a diaper, the woman cooking a meal, the person changing a tire for a neighbor, and someone feeding stray cats, [are] all touching the world for good."

Father Breighner writes that people often ask him how they can know whether they are doing God's will. If he doesn't have a lot of time to spend with the person in conversation or counseling, he says, "I usually quote a dictum from the 12-step programs: 'Do the next right thing.'

"If we fill a need," the priest goes on, "correct a wrong, lend a hand, speak words of encouragement, in short, do the good thing for those nearest us, we will be doing God's will."

Whatever you believe or don't believe when it comes to religion, let me say this in a language that each of us can embrace: We live the best life within reach *every time* we touch another person's life with kindness. As your loved one's caregiver, perhaps you underestimate the great value of small good deeds, done daily. Your simple acts of giving comfort and aid, showing respect, and practicing kindness *do* matter. They matter a lot.

You're Not a Bad Person Because You're Exhausted or Just Need a Life of Your Own

I was trying to manage an unmanageable situation. What on earth is it like for others? I clearly still needed help—and I was a psychiatric nurse who had worked with hospitalized patients for 26 years!
—Cindy J., RN, BSN

In the stories that follow, we see the challenges faced when a daughter's physical and emotional resources wear thin as she travels significant distances to oversee the care of her widowed mother and developmentally disabled sister. Challenges aplenty, however, also confront the next family, whose impaired elderly loved one lives just next door, in an apartment adjoining the home. Shared here are the fascinatingly different perspectives of two uniquely challenging situations.

CINDY'S CHALLENGE: LONG-DISTANCE CAREGIVING

For many years, Cindy was among the 15 percent of long-distance caregivers in America who struggle to solve problems and provide an elderly loved one with family support. As often as once a month, she traveled from Maryland to New York. In Buffalo her developmentally disabled sister, Janet, lived in a group home in the suburbs, while her mother lived nearby—five years in an assisted living apartment, two years in a memory care facility, and another year in a nursing home. The years of caring for her sister are over, with no regrets, while the emotional challenges of caring for her mother are still playing out, with painful twists and turns over the years, and have yet to find their ending.

Devoting countless three-day weekends to caring for them, she took her sister to visit their mother and individually or together took them to lunch, shopping, and to dinner. It helped that a staff member at the group home took Cindy's sister to visit their mother at least once a week. Until their conditions worsened, this arrangement was workable.

Cindy's mother had lived in her own home for six years after becoming a widow, but she felt isolated there following the deaths of her sisters and many friends. "Maybe if I hadn't been a nurse, I would not have started investigating assisted living arrangements as soon as I did," Cindy explained. It was a wise decision and lengthened her mother's years of enjoying a quality life. "Mother's apartment was very nice. She had her belongings, made new friends, and loved it. She felt more comfortable and less anxious."

Cindy's brother sold the family home and managed their parents' resources well, she told me, but "we went through a shocking amount of money over the next eight years. We thought this assisted living apartment was her last stop, but that was not to be."

When Cindy's brother died of renal cancer at the age of 62, "it was so painful that our mother never spoke of it, and [losing him] seemed to be the straw that broke the camel's back." There were some early signs of Alzheimer's disease. By the time their mother entered her late 80s, Cindy saw that her mother repeated herself often and forgot things, including leaving food cooking on the burner. The stove in her kitchenette had to be disconnected, but the microwave sufficed for a while.

Uncharacteristically, Cindy's mother began to plead, "I'm so afraid! I'm so afraid!" She started folding up little pieces of Kleenex, rolled up in little squares. "Cindy, are you sure you know your way home? I'm afraid," her mother would say again and again. To this mental health nurse, taking the next step became a matter of urgency.

Cindy found a "wonderful" memory care center, "a beautiful facility with an amazing social worker. It was a good facility meant to care for patients with Alzheimer's disease. The residents were free to walk about in a safe environment that was not too restrictive."

The transition from assisted living, however, was difficult for all concerned. It isn't possible to convince a person who has lost her decision-making capacity (competency) that leaving her apartment is in her best interest. Although necessary to provide an advanced level of care for her mother's condition, a facility that looks "beautiful" to a family member can represent a puzzling and possibly frightening change. It was gut-wrenchingly sad for Cindy to hear her mother ask, "Why do I have to leave here? Did I do something wrong? What did I do that they don't want me here any longer?"

Making a move also can accelerate the already expected progression of a person's Alzheimer's disease. "I'd bring my sister to the memory care center when I visited my mother, who was getting more and more confused," Cindy told me. "She became more cognitively impaired than Janet, my sister who had cerebral palsy and could only read at the first-grade level."

"There were times in the nursing home, when I was not happy, when they didn't treat her with the dignity she deserved," Cindy recalled. "Someone would lose my mother's glasses or not put in her hearing aid. My mother would have a rosary but it became lost and would end up in the room of another confused patient. The staff in this center didn't care about any of that: it was absolutely outrageous! We bought another set of hearing aids and I would just go out and get another rosary, but some things—like missing photographs—were irreplaceable. I was there frequently, and, when the staff members saw me often, things were sometimes better."

They celebrated her ninetieth birthday, but the elderly woman was in sharp decline. "My mother's personality became so different. She would say things that were mean or rude. She was never like that and would have been mortified had she known."

Her mother had a gallbladder attack and had to be hospitalized. The doctor wanted to operate, but Cindy would have none of it: "They were not doing surgery on an already frail, elderly person!" As a nurse, she knew her mother would probably survive the surgery but likely would be confused and frightened, lie in recovery with a respirator, and awaken with no idea of where she was or what had happened or the reason for the surgery. Later, a less invasive medical procedure was done on an outpatient basis that gave her mother the needed relief.

Deeply troubled, she recalled how "the quality of my mother's life vanished in the last 18 months of her life." Cindy later told her own children, "If I'm very old and progressively cognitively impaired, don't decide to do major surgery! Let me die a natural death."

When Cindy's mother was ready to leave the hospital, she was no longer eligible for the memory care center because, even with a walker, she couldn't walk the distance considered to be "ambulatory," from her room to the dining room. The hospitalist (doctor in charge at the hospital) told Cindy that her mother had to go to a nursing home.

"I'd left my job flying back and forth so often that I couldn't do it anymore. With my amazing husband's support, I decided to bring my mother back to our home," which by this time was in South Carolina. "At that point, Mom could still respond to my being there and she would be a lot more calm. That's why I thought she'd be better going back with me, because I could comfort her."

Almost as soon as her mother had a bedroom in South Carolina, it got to be too much. "Being in my home was not comforting. It was so difficult to see my mother deteriorate to the point that she did, and I was having a hard time finding caregivers who would reliably come to relieve me. When I went to a local United Fund support group for caregivers," Cindy vividly remembers, "I was so emotionally devastated that all I could do was cry. I couldn't contribute. It was hard to let myself need help when I'd always been the helper."

Fortunately, Cindy did finally allow herself to be on the receiving end of the compassion, understanding, and support of the kind she had been giving to others for most of her adult life. The group members, also caregivers of impaired elderly loved ones, understood her pain and gave her a safe haven to express it.

Cindy had known her mom as "such a dear, good, and kind person." Fearing that people who had never known her mother would see only the dementia and not the person she used to be, Cindy didn't allow her South Carolina friends to see her mother.

After several weeks of "my attention revolving around taking care of Mother, including when we were up all night," Cindy knew that she had to find a nursing home. "My husband was incredible to assist me, but having her live in our home was very stressful. Truthfully, because I had done so much inpatient nursing, I had thought I could handle it—but nothing seemed to relieve my mother's confusion, anxiety, and agitation. I understood medicines, problems in elderly people, and what to look out for, but I *still* couldn't do it."

In the words of Cindy's friend, a woman who had experienced the tragic death of a young son and other great losses, "There are some things that are so bad that you just can't make them good." In my personal experience, too, and my work with grieving people, I know there are times when we are utterly powerless to save or protect our loved ones. This is simply part of the human condition, something we have no choice but to accept.

She decided to find her mother a nursing home in Buffalo. She didn't want to send her back to the one she had found so unacceptable. Back in Buffalo, where Cindy had always had a place to stay overnight with Alice, her dearest friend since childhood, she could resume taking her sister to visit their mother. "By the grace of God, we somehow got my mother back to New York and I found a facility that I felt comfortable with. My mother was very agitated and would call out in ways disruptive to the unit and painful for everybody. Sometimes she would calm down if I sat with her or she would doze off. Sometimes it didn't help at all that I was there."

Now when she flew in from South Carolina, Cindy stayed two weeks at a time. She is grateful for the medical professionals who listened to her concerns and tried to relieve her mother's pain and anxiety. "In all my experience working with doctors, I was very clear that you had to be very careful in an effort to avoid giving antipsychotic medicines like Haldol, if at all possible." Sometimes there may be no choice, if the patient with dementia is delusional or hallucinating. But, as often happens, the Haldol added to her mother's confusion and agitation. The antidepressant and antianxiety drugs that were prescribed were more helpful. Unfortunately, nothing helped to completely calm her mother. It was agonizing to watch.

Cindy's close friendship with Alice was "life saving." Always being able to return to Alice's house for respite after a hard day at the nursing home gave Cindy a place to talk over the ordeal or (as she often preferred) to escape it. "My friendship with Alice had such incredible meaning to me," she told me.

Cindy's sister, Janet, was 66 and her health was failing. "I would stay six hours, give my mother her meal, just sit with her, then go get my sister and we three would sit together."

When their mother would say something really unpleasant, it was difficult for Janet to understand because of her developmental disabilities. "It was strange to her that our mother was so different. Janet never expressed being distressed or dismayed and would always have asked, 'Are we going to see Mom?' If my sister said anything showing too much distress, I would have stopped taking her to the nursing home."

When their mother passed away at the age of 92, "family came from all over the country, my sister went to the funeral, sat at the cemetery, and came back with the family for dinner. She told me, 'I don't have a mother anymore.' Janet loved being with all of her family, including nieces and nephews. What a blessing it was that my sister got to have such a good time. Sixteen days later she died."

Few Regrets and Many Lessons Learned

Cindy is 68 years old now. It has been nearly 10 years since her mother and sister died. "I don't regret doing any of those things," she told me. "There's nothing better than making a difference in someone's life. I'm glad I had that experience. I was the baby in the family. I never imagined being the caretaker."

She regrets only that her mother had that period of time in the nursing home when she seemed to feel "tortured" and wishes "so much that I would have gotten hospice care so maybe Mother's life would have ended more peacefully, perhaps months earlier [with the pain medication often administered in hospice care]." As a nurse, Cindy had seen medication bring comfort to hospice patients as they approached the end of their lives.

Cindy wondered, "Did I do everything I could do? I loved her. I didn't contact hospice because, as a nurse, I thought the social worker in the nursing home would know when to talk to me about hospice." She wishes she'd have listened to her own inner voice and spoken with the nursing home doctor to advocate for hospice care.

Cindy struggled with feelings of guilt over the various ways she couldn't do more for her mother, including having been on an airplane on her way to her mother and not there in time to be with her when she died. Her best friend Alice's words of support were spot on: "I was living in the same house with my mom, and even then wasn't with her when she died." Alice also found just the right question to ask: "And what would your loving mother say to you about *all that?*"

"She'd say that I did the best that I could do," Cindy replied. "She'd say, 'You're a good daughter. It's okay. I had a good life.'"

Sometimes we just have to accept the limits of our control over fateful circumstances and events, as difficult as that may be. "If I had known then what I know now," we have to remind ourselves, "I'd have done things differently." Like Cindy and Alice, I also wish I could have been with my dear mother when she died. Having stayed with her day and night at the hospice for several days, I was across town visiting my dad in the hospital when the phone call came. I'm also sorry that I couldn't be there to hold the hand of my grandmother in Oklahoma, my brother in Oregon, and my friend Dorris in North Carolina as they passed away. But what I do know—as firmly as I know my own name—is that all the love that we share with our parents, grandparents, siblings, spouses, and other loved ones is *love that will never die.* What we need to do is call to mind our loving memories, learn to forgive our own and our loved ones' failings, and let go of whatever distracting or menacing thoughts would rob us of recalling the precious, fond experiences we shared.

Reflecting back, Cindy continued, "The baby in the family was meant to have these responsibilities. In the long run, I was the right person, the only one who went into a medical field. Sometimes the only choice we are left with is to make that decision to ask ourselves, 'How will I grow from this experience?'"

Brought up in a Catholic household, "I wasn't a practicing Catholic for a long time," she explained, because of certain teachings she still doesn't agree with. "But the church is part of my life now. Through the power of rituals and the liturgy, I'm able to attend to the messages better than when I was younger. As I've gotten older, my religious upbringing has gotten more important. My husband is Jewish and we celebrate both Christian and Jewish holidays, both equally meaningful."

Clearly for Cindy, especially in recent years, "faith helps provide a certain amount of calm and comfort." My hope for *you*, as the reader of this book, is that you will find whatever is your own spiritual or secular path to finding a sense of peace, whether it is through rituals of thanksgiving, prayer, meditation, yoga, nature's beauty, service to others, the arts, inspirational readings or uplifting music, or loving relationships.

For Cindy, a powerful part of her mother's legacy is the way that their love lives on through a shared ritual. "My mother said the rosary every morning after she woke up," Cindy explained, as sweet tears fell. "I have her rosary now, and she has passed that spirituality on to me. There is tremendous solace that I get from holding my mother's rosary and saying those prayers."

Cindy strongly believes that "things happen for a reason. We are meant to learn from experiences that can make each of us a better person, more able to help other people." She realizes now how much pain caregivers live with and how greatly they need to be helped to relieve that pain. "Being able to talk to people who were not judgmental and could handle my sharing the sad, hard parts of caring for my mother has made me a more attentive and understanding listener."

Throughout her caregiving years, Cindy learned "that there are a lot of amazing people out there who can help." Especially comforting are the opportunities to talk with other women who also had a close relationship with their mothers, she explains. "It's meaningful to share a recognition, after you lose that person, that certain things live on in you that were part of your mother, [traits and qualities] you see in yourself."

Cindy has discovered that "to be in nature helps me, too. I'd always been a city girl until we moved to this little seaside community in South Carolina. I get absorbed in the walks I take, looking at the water and loving the smell of it. I'd never realized until I retired here how much pleasure and healing I find in bird watching and gardening. I didn't know I was such a nature girl."

Plenty of Reasons to Be Thankful

"I realize," Cindy continued, "how fortunate I am to have the family I have. I know I was loved unconditionally, and not everybody has that. When I see other family dynamics, not all parents are as loving, not everyone had a big brother who could look out for them. I'm lucky I had the sister I had. Despite her disabilities, she was a gentle, nice person to be around. She didn't complain. People wanted to work with her in her setting. When we would go to her group home, she would jump out of her chair when she saw us."

Cindy is also thankful that "my mother and my sister showed me how to be empathic to people's frailties and disabilities. I saw that my sister had disabilities, and I saw how my mother was so devoted to Janet and gave her a good quality of life. Throughout her childhood, Janet was surrounded by family, was loved, attended special education schools, and until just days before she died was still taking part in family events."

There was in her family of birth, Cindy realizes, "an acceptance and a valuing of individual differences, whether people were mentally disabled, gay, a different religion or race. My parents demonstrated understanding and respect for other people. They respected other people's religions or secular beliefs and believed that God's love is shared with all of humanity."

She is thankful for the daughter and son she loves dearly from her first marriage and is thankful that her present husband of 26 years, Barry, is "such a good guy. He is an accepting person who extends himself to others, is a loving father to his children, and he has developed a good relationship with my adult children as well. Barry is the most likeable person you'd ever want to meet," she says proudly.

Nothing is ever perfect. For Cindy, her husband, and their blended family of four children living in three distant states, there are financial issues to resolve and decisions to make regarding some potentially significant challenges ahead. As a couple, they have managed many life transitions, crises, and troubles in the past. Hopefully, in the near future, they will figure out how to plan for their own late adult life. "We need to be thoughtful about what the next move will be," she says. "What my parents saved and my brother invested for them was well beyond what most people can afford, and certainly beyond the resources Barry and I can provide, if our children have to arrange our care in late life."

Cindy regrets that she thought it impossible to start any financial planning when she was a young nurse in the 1980s. She was a single parent then and couldn't imagine how it could be possible to set aside money for old age. Cindy also wishes that she and Barry had looked into getting long-term care insurance when it might have been affordable, in their late fifties. "Fortunately my daughter and son, in their 40s, are planning earlier and more wisely for their own retirements," she says.

"Here's What I Want My Children to Remember When I Am Old"

Reflecting on the future's uncertainties, Cindy has come to think of growing older in a way more protective of her loved ones: "On the one hand, I can say I did everything in my power to give my mother the best care that she could receive, but I want to say to my own children that such sacrifice on their part is not what I want for myself."

With an increasing sense of the importance of having this conversation more than once, so that it is clearly understood, Cindy says, "I am telling my adult children that, when the time comes, we can't afford and I don't need a really nice facility with bells and whistles." Acknowledging that her financial situation is unlike her mother's, continues Cindy, "I will say to my daughter and son, 'Just find a place where you feel they are giving good care. The so-called beautiful facility doesn't necessarily do that. I also don't expect and don't have the money for you to hire people. The most important thing is that you show up. *Just come visit as often as you can.*'"

Cindy and her husband "never anticipated that we are living in our forever home," she says, "but until the housing market improves, we would lose just too much money to sell now." The yard work and larger house are still manageable, but they realize that it's important to downsize and not wait until fate puts the burden of making such decisions on their children's shoulders.

"I wish we could do the old fashioned thing and just live in the same city as our children, but that's not possible. We know we have to make a change," Cindy says emphatically, "but we are *done* with the snow and cold weather! We are not going backward and moving back to Maryland [where his children live] or going to ice-cold Minnesota [where her daughter lives], and California [where her son lives] is too expensive."

On the other hand, Cindy remembers all too vividly the ordeal of "having to take at least two airplanes to Buffalo, which was costly and added a huge amount of travel time to those countless trips." Each of Cindy and Barry's four children from their first marriages, when they come to visit, already cope with that same airline complication and expense.

Their plan for making it easier for their children to look after them as older adults, is to remain in the warm South but move near a city large enough to have an airport with direct flights from Baltimore, Minneapolis, and San Francisco. Cindy wants to make it workable and reasonable to repeat her request, *"Just come visit as often as you can."*

MICHELLE CARTER: "TO SAY IT WAS CHAOS, IS REALLY AN UNDERSTATEMENT"

Caring for your spouse, your children, and yourself can sometimes "get lost" as you approach the challenge of caring for your own or your spouse's aging parents. That's what happened to Michelle Carter, who took on the challenge of having her in-laws live with the couple and their two young daughters. She started out with kind and generous intentions, only to find herself dealing with consequences she never imagined.

After Michelle and I had started our interviews, she went home and wrote down her recollections as to how she had gotten into this situation:

> You won't believe this but the whole idea of moving in with my in-laws was my idea! I saw the writing on the wall. My husband's sister, Roxanne, lived in another state, and, additionally, she was emotionally distant from her parents. LeRoy was spending more and more time over at my in-laws' house helping my mother-in-law with her husband, who was recently diagnosed with Alzheimer's disease. They had lived in their house for over 50 years with many repairs and updates needing to be done to it. My mother-in-law couldn't manage the house and take care of my father-in-law. There was no way she was going to go into an assisted living arrangement or send her husband into a facility by himself.
>
> LeRoy and I had a two-year-old daughter and lived in a very small house.

We had started to look for a bigger house to accommodate our growing family. I kept thinking that, wherever we moved, my husband's parents would end up living with us, so I made the proposal to my husband to go into a house together with his parents. At that time, five years into our marriage, I felt I had a nice relationship with LeRoy's parents. I also saw the love that LeRoy felt for his parents and they for him. LeRoy took the idea to his mother to sell both our houses and find a house with an in-law suite or the capability of adding an in-law suite to the house. She was thrilled that we would want to move in together and I think relieved that there was an answer to her dilemma. My father-in-law's illness was so progressed that there was no discussion with him about selling the house (that he had built) and moving out. My mother-in-law was involved in the whole process of house hunting and had full say over what house we would own. There was one particular house that we put a bid on and didn't get that my mother-in-law and I were very sad about. We both loved that house, but the timing wasn't right. LeRoy and I ended up selling our house and moving in with my in-laws for three months while still looking for a house to buy.

Meanwhile I was pregnant with our second, Kalya. It took a total of a year to find a house that could meet our needs, everyone agreed on, and fit into our budget.

—Michelle

She was nearly nine months pregnant with Kalya, and Katrina was three years old, when she, LeRoy, and his parents moved into a house large enough for them all once the renovations added on an adjoining apartment for LeRoy's folks. His father's Alzheimer's disease was progressing, and an agency caregiver needed to be hired to help. The big house had a two-car garage with an already finished upstairs bedroom. It was ideal for adding a downstairs living room/bedroom, full bath, small kitchen, and laundry. There would be front and back doors and windows, and a wide door between the apartment and the main house. Everything would be wheelchair accessible.

Just as most construction projects seem to take longer than expected, LeRoy's parents ended up staying in the family room shared by everyone, for a long *three months*. This was complicated by the fact that LeRoy's 81-year-old father became wheelchair bound three days after they all moved in together. Sharing one house was made all the more challenging by the fact that his 79-year-old mother, Michelle realized belatedly, was "a very difficult person in her dealings with other women," most especially LeRoy's sister, and a major challenge for Michelle.

"It was very stressful," Michelle continued. "We had to carry two mortgages until we sold his parents' house. Meanwhile, there was 50 years' worth of stuff to sort through before we could sell it. At home, I had a newborn and a little girl recently potty trained, one kitchen, one laundry room—and a mother-in-law who wanted to be the one in charge! It seemed like LeRoy was always at his job or working at his folks' house, and I was constantly cooking and cleaning up for everyone." Michelle, swamped with childcare, kept trying to cope with her frequently complaining, ever-present, and rather bossy mother-in-law.

Initially, more than a dozen of her father-in-law's paid caregivers came and left, Michelle explained, "because my mother-in-law said one after another wouldn't listen to her. She was so difficult to please that some of the caregivers from the elder care agency didn't want to come back, and, about the others, my mother-in-law would say, 'we need to try someone else.'

"It was terrible," Michelle remembers, with depressing clarity. "Uprooted from her home, my mother-in-law was completely stressed out." LeRoy thought Michelle was exaggerating when she tried to tell him that his mother added tension to the house, much of the day. Her mother-in-law's "poor me" attitude and seeming effort to have all of the household's attention focused on her, good or bad, was wearing on Michelle's ordinarily upbeat personality, and her generous spirit was taking a hit, too.

"I was on the downstairs sofa, breastfeeding my baby, covered up and every-thing, when LeRoy's mother kept shooting me a disgusted stare, like I was doing something horrible. LeRoy's father, on the other side of the room, was too impaired to realize what was going on, and the lady who was his caretaker also didn't seem to notice or care. Eventually, I was made to feel so uncomfort-able by my mother-in-law's obvious disapproval that I started feeding Kalya only upstairs. This was inconvenient because Kalya never would take a bottle and was wanting to be fed. One time, when I descended the stairs after breast-feeding, my mother-in-law said she'd been *'waiting down here for a long time,'* wanting to go to the store, but she 'didn't want to leave three-year-old Katrina *alone.*' Well, my father-in-law's caregiver was right there, and I was only up-stairs. When I asked why didn't she just call up the stairway and say she was leaving to run an errand, my mother-in-law answered that she thought I was sleeping—in the middle of the afternoon!"

While Michelle already had an inkling that her mother-in-law's tendency was to be happiest when others focused their attention on her, "until we all moved in together, I had no idea that she had a cruel streak." Complaining to LeRoy, Michelle said, "I need more help around here." His mother, overhearing this, answered, "*I'll* start helping when *she* does!"

On most occasions, LeRoy defended his mother, but this was a time when he saw what his wife had been trying to tell him. Michelle recalled that LeRoy actually yelled at his mother, "Don't talk about my wife like that! I know that's not true."

His mother, answering in anger, threatened, "I'm going to call my lawyers and get out of this!"

Remembering another time when LeRoy had a taste of the sour medicine his mother had been spooning out in large doses for her, Michelle continued, "LeRoy was mad because we have hardwood floors and his mother kept moving a chair that had already gouged the floor."

When he said something to her, his mother dispensed the overdose: "These floors are mine, too, and I can scratch them if I want to!"

Unfortunately, however, "almost always LeRoy gave his mother the benefit of the doubt," Michelle recalled. "Every time my mother-in-law got mad at me, she would go out and buy my three-year-old a Barbie doll, and I would *never* have bought a three-year-old a Barbie doll."

When Michelle complained to LeRoy, more often than not, he would say, "I'm sure you're reading into it, that she didn't mean it that way."

A good thing was that LeRoy's dad—even with dementia—had a personality that was a study in contrasts as compared with LeRoy's mother. "He was the kindest, gentlest man to the end," Michelle fondly recalled. "The only time he'd get upset was if the paid caretaker was dressing him, but he was never mean. I'd walk into the room, and my father-in-law would have no idea who I was, but he'd say, 'Hello! How are you? Don't you look pretty!'"

After they moved into their own apartment, LeRoy's mother made her own breakfast and lunch while the helper fed LeRoy's father. Michelle continued to make and serve dinner for everyone, when the couple's paid helper was about to leave. His mother cut up her husband's food and fed him at the dining table in the big house. "She was mostly pretty patient with him in his frail years," Michelle recalls. LeRoy and his mother took care of getting his father to the bathroom and into bed every night.

The frail, elderly man's last paid caregiver was a woman named Margie, who took such good care of him that LeRoy's mother, afraid Margie might go work for someone else, started giving her expensive gifts and money for car repairs. "Then when my father-in-law died, just two years after we combined our homes," Michelle told me, "Margie kept calling my mother-in-law to say how upset she was over his death. She repeatedly told her own sad stories and asked for money. My mother-in-law was giving away hundreds and hundreds of dollars."

This was one of the times when Michelle's husband saw immediately what was going on. Something similar had happened a couple of years earlier, when his parents were back at their home. A helper had talked his mother into pre-paying the helper's husband $800 for lawn work, had stolen a blank check from the house, and had used it to pay her own $1,000 rent. LeRoy's mother had then refused to prosecute.

"This time, LeRoy's mother asked us to answer the phone," Michelle recalled. "When Margie kept calling, we made up excuses for his mother and said she was asleep or had gone out."

A Generous Grandmother

"There were happy times," Michelle remembers. "My mother-in-law and I got along for periods of time. For the next five years after LeRoy's dad died, his mother kept more to herself and came over less. She went out more and seemed to enjoy a sense of freedom, had friends and could still drive, but she was never good about picking up that phone and making plans." But what she *did* do, to her own benefit and for the good of the family, was spend quality time gardening with Michelle and enjoying activities with Kalya and Katrina. "Since my mother-in-law had a good eye for creating an attractive flower garden, I could ask for her advice on where to put the plants she bought, and we kind of bonded working together in the yard."

The girls often liked to go to Grandma's apartment to play with their dolls, which was something their grandma loved to do with them. They also played cards and other games, worked puzzles and read stories together. During many of those visits to Grandma's apartment next door, Michelle disapproved of how much television the girls got to watch, but the children liked it.

The little girls' favorite activity was to dig into Grandma's chest of drawers to find scarves, sweaters, and costume jewelry for dress-up play. Occasionally Kalya and Katrina put on puppet shows for everyone back at the big house. Attended by their parents and Grandma in the audience, a favorite family event was a "fashion show," something the girls came up with on their own and performed, wearing Grandma's clothes and jewelry from that special drawer. Michelle still remembers the happy look on her husband's face as he watched his mother laugh and enjoy Kalya and Katrina's special performance.

Michelle's mother-in-law has always been generous with her grandchildren in financial ways. She paid the entire way for her daughter Roxanne's (now grown) children to attend private school and helped with their college and recreational expenses, and she is helping LeRoy's children as well by contributing to the tuition for Kalya and Katrina's schooling and also to their college fund.

Passive-Aggressive Behavior

Michelle at times has wondered whether her mother-in-law's financial generosity has come with an unwelcome emotional price to be paid by her sister-in-law and Michelle and LeRoy's family, too. Did her mother-in-law think that giving so generously to the four grandchildren entitled her to speak freely words so often unkind or dismissive of others' feelings?

"My mother-in-law has had a habit of saying and doing passive-aggressive things," Michelle told me, "but not when LeRoy was here. For example, when LeRoy's sister was coming to visit from Virginia, she bought all of Roxanne's favorite junk foods before she arrived, then when Roxanne ate it, my mother-in-law was quick to admonish her daughter: 'No wonder you can't lose weight! Your small frame can't handle all the extra weight you carry!'

"This is how she treats her daughter," Michelle explains. "She is always finding fault with Roxanne and bringing up mean, hurtful things to say. But LeRoy is her golden boy; she is quick to forgive *him*."

Michelle describes herself as a "very health-oriented" parent. While she acknowledges that many grandparents like to "spoil" their grandchildren with sweets, "that doesn't work when you live in the same house." Kalya and Katrina, now ages 10 and 13, when younger, "would go next door where their grandmother had desserts at all times of the day. They would eat cookies at 11:00 in the morning, their grandmother not minding that it was before lunch, then the girls would barely eat lunch."

She would explain to her mother-in-law that "my girls have a small appetite" and say she wanted her children to have lunch and only have dessert after they'd had a good meal. "Sometimes she was responsive and stopped giving the kids sweets before a mealtime, even though my husband grew up in a house where sweets were available any time of day. But at other times," Michelle laments, "she really lashed out at me."

"You aren't being a kind mother! You're just depriving them," her mother-in-law would say.

"It was like that," Michelle remembers well, "when I was trying to get my daughters to clean their rooms, or pick up their toys before a play date. She would say I was being too hard on them and overly harsh. For having to pick up their toys?"

How This Daughter-in-Law Has Survived

"For the first two years, when I was around my family and friends, all I did was complain. I still have so many bad memories. We had extra money from the sale of our house but we put that into remodeling, so money has been tight for a long time. Recently, I told LeRoy, 'When you mother is gone, I want to sell the house. Half of the furniture here is hers. I never felt that this house was mine.' "

To cope with the stress, keep her marriage intact, and continue to enjoy life with her husband and children, Michelle describes the activities that have sustained her: regular exercise and fitness workouts, part-time employment outside the home, close friendships, and lifelong learning. "I have to make exercise a priority and not feel guilty or selfish about it. I have to do this for myself and for the benefit of everyone else. I am a runner. I work out. I do yoga. I let it all out. I have learned to put things in perspective. I don't dwell on it. What good would that do?"

For a while, Michelle confessed, "I felt like I hated my mother-in-law, and I asked myself, 'How am I ever going to like this person again?' Finally, I realized that how she was treating me didn't have anything much to do with me. She was treating me in these [hurtful] ways because of *her*, not because of *me*. I also decided that my husband doesn't need me to be complaining about her every night when he comes home. I finally just had to let my anger go. I realized that there's no reason for hanging on to anger; it doesn't do you any good."

Except for the first year after her Kalya was born, the year when everyone moved into the big house together, Michelle has always had at least one part-time job. Married almost 17 years, she was coordinating a sexual violence hotline and working on a master's degree when she got pregnant with Katrina, 14 years ago. Since then, Michelle worked retail part time for a jewelry store then became and still works as the store's diamond inventory keeper. She studied and became a certified personal trainer, then took another course to become a master gardener. "Three years ago," Michelle told me, "it was another wonderful outlet, when I went back to college part time to finish my master's degree. So many stay-at-home moms only talk about their kids and have nothing else. I didn't want to be that mom." She is looking for full-time work now.

Michelle says she has "a great network of friends, including a best friend" she is able to confide in, who lives in a nearby neighborhood. Her daughters, now 10 and 13, are up late at night these days, leaving Michelle to yearn for private time with LeRoy. She rues the fact that her husband is "always working so hard" and complains that the two of them rarely get even a day or two away for a holiday. "He will come home from a long day and could sit down to eat with us, but he goes straight to her apartment to visit his mother. He truly loves our daughters and I know he loves me, but he's not even with us when he's home. I want to say, 'Think about our daughters and how much you're missing out on.'"

Self-talk is helpful, Michelle explains. "After all these years, it can't last much longer. Then I'll get my husband back. He doesn't 'get' it, though. He gives me a compliment, which signals to me that he wants sex. But we don't even talk and spend time together, so how are we going to have sex? I can't not spend time with him and then feel like making love. But he's a guy. For him, sex is an outlet. I can be mean to him, but part of that is all about my feeling resentful. *I don't want it to be too late to save our marriage.*"

For Now, Michelle's Decision about Her Mother's and Her Own Old Age

Michelle is 46. Her mother is 71, just ten years older than Michelle's husband. Not long ago, LeRoy said, "*Your* mom could always come stay with us."

Although Michelle says that her mom is the dearest person she knows, her response to LeRoy was, "I love you and I know it would be nothing like it was. I just don't want to go through that again."

She knows that her mother-in-law "got to see her grandchildren come visit and play cards with her. They brought her a lot of joy, but that's not enough, and sitting with her in recent years is more of a chore for the girls now," Michelle says. "You need to live your own life. I look at my mother-in-law and I say, 'That will not be me.' She was pretty much a shut-in for the last six years. Her doctor would tell her that she needed to get out and walk, which she didn't do. Maybe it would have been different if she had acclimated and been around people her own age."

Today, Michelle feels strongly about one thing: "I know that I will not do this to my children. I will go into a facility while I'm still healthy and make friends and make that my home."

"This Is When It Gets Really Bad"

About two years ago, when her health was failing, LeRoy's mother repeated the process of hiring and firing six or eight caregivers or having them quit. At 89, she finally found an agency caregiver she liked very much, a woman who became her companion and aide. Afraid of losing this caregiver to another job and unbeknownst to her family, from the ages of 89 to 91 (when she was still writing checks), LeRoy's mother paid the agency caregiver for ten extra hours of work every week—hours that she wasn't working! This was discovered when LeRoy's mother had to be hospitalized for a few weeks, and Michelle and LeRoy found the checkbook. "Oh my gosh," Michelle exclaimed, "this woman had totally been ripping off my mother-in-law and was overpaid by as much as ten thousand dollars!" It was also discovered that the caregiver, "on the sly," had talked the elderly woman into hiring *the caregiver's mother* to do weekend work. Not reporting this to the agency employing the caregiver was in violation of their contract.

The hospitalization had taken place after several months of increasingly frequent, nighttime psychotic episodes, causing extreme disruptions at the Carters' house. "Last year, my mother-in-law started hearing voices," Michelle explained. "There were tormenting voices saying they were going to come get her, or that she was a terrible person and was going to hell. She also heard good, sweet voices, but the bad ones were terribly frightening and outnumbered the good."

Michelle and LeRoy almost never got away for a vacation, not even for a few days. "His mother was always nervous when we weren't there next door," Michelle continued, near tears. On one of those rare occasions, Michelle hired two college-age sisters from the neighborhood to babysit the girls and look after LeRoy's mother. "We were only going to be gone for two nights, and the first night at 3:00 a.m. we got a call that his mother had smelled gas in the house, thought the oven was left on, and—instead of waking anyone—had used her Life Alert to call the fire department!" That was in April. It happened again in July. And it happened again in August, "when LeRoy and I awoke in the middle of the night to a police officer coming up the stairs toward our bedroom!"

The officer yelled up, "We got a call that voices were heard in the house. After talking to this lady [LeRoy's mother, who was standing near the open front door, next to another policeman], we thought maybe you were okay."

"Luckily the officers didn't have their guns drawn," Michelle sighed, "but we were startled."

Increasingly impaired, LeRoy's mother "kept having these spells of hearing frightening voices in the night and pushing her Life Alert button. At least five times, over a period of several months, either the police department or fire department was dispatched to the house at odd hours of the night." Of course, because of her dementia and the fact that the antipsychotic medicine she takes helps only to a degree, there is no malice involved. At the age of 91, she is no longer mentally competent.

After returning from her stay in a psychiatric hospital, things improved but LeRoy and Michelle needed to hire round-the-clock care, two 12-hour caregiver shifts. "My mother-in-law's long-term care insurance only pays $100 a day," Michelle explained, with concern. "So in just one week at $20 an hour, the cost was $3,360—and $2,660 of that was not covered by the insurance. The cost was outrageous!" So they could cut that cost in half, LeRoy set up a bed in the living room, kept the door ajar to his mother's apartment in case she woke up at night, and started sleeping there. Michelle, understandably, was beginning to be pushed to her limits. "I wondered when I would ever get my husband back," she told me.

Recently there was a fall. With a broken hip came surgery. Michelle's mother-in-law for the last three or four weeks has been in a rehabilitation facility, a period Michelle says could have been a "thrilling break" allowing for more time together. Unfortunately, "LeRoy goes there after work and stays several hours, even when she is sleeping. When he has been there most of the day on a weekend, when he gets up to leave, his mother says, 'What? You're leaving?'"

Regrettably, instead of finally having the delight of a peaceful house all to themselves as a married couple with two daughters, Michelle says, "LeRoy's sister has come from Virginia and is staying in the in-law apartment. She comes over first thing in the morning with her laptop. In our stone house, the only place with Internet reception is at the dining room table!" Much like her mother, Roxanne often talks nonstop and seems to need everyone's attention. "Then when Roxanne goes to visit at the rehab center," Michelle tells me, "she sends a stream of texts to LeRoy, who is busy at work all day long, giving him a play-by-play account of events at the rehab center. She tells him how their mother insists that everyone with whom she has shared a room is plotting against her, and that another patient keeps calling their mother a 'whore.' Then when LeRoy doesn't answer his sister's texts," Michelle sighs, "Roxanne texts *me* to ask why isn't LeRoy answering her texts."

LeRoy's sister had a relationship with her mother that was so contentious throughout her growing up years that it has remained troubled. Over many years, Roxanne has rarely even visited her mother. As Michelle sees it, "Roxanne is now trying to atone by being here constantly while her mother is recovering from hip surgery. But, as always, she stays a while then, for months at a time, Roxanne leaves all the caregiving to us. Now she is asking lots of very personal, intrusive questions about our financial situation, implying we've been taking money for ourselves from LeRoy's mother!

"When LeRoy comes home late at night now, Roxanne leaps to her feet and meets her brother at the door, regaling him with the day's events related to visiting their mother!" Michelle resents the fact that she can't have her husband alone, after he was at work all day, then went straight to see his mother at the rehabilitation facility.

After three weeks of this, Michelle recently said to her sister-in-law, "Why don't you take a break from visiting your mother for a couple of days and come back next week? That will be good for you, plus LeRoy and I can have some time for a break, too."

Roxanne, outwardly angry on hearing this, took offense. Later, LeRoy scolded Michelle, saying, "I can't believe you said that to Roxanne! I feel the same way but I would never have said it!"

This Couple Needs a "Zone of Protection"

What Michelle and LeRoy didn't do—eleven years ago—and haven't done since, was establish a "zone of protection" for themselves as a couple and on behalf of their own growing family. It is so easy to slip into early habits as an individual or married couple, including patterns like putting your parents' needs ahead of your own. Loving and honoring one's spouse, parent, or sibling when that person is elderly and ill, impaired or becoming frail is a good and honorable, natural thing to do. Of course, there are times when loving someone means that we temporarily sacrifice our own and our immediate family's well being. It's just that patterns are hard to break. We need to know that not only is it okay to make decisions that enable us to take good care of ourselves; it is *necessary* to set certain boundaries so that self-care becomes an essential part of becoming a kind and effective caregiver for what is often a long road to travel.

Trouble Ahead?

"LeRoy's mother guilt trips him," Michelle realizes, "and so does his sister. They manipulate him and take advantage of his loyalty and good nature." Sadly, as I listen to Michelle through more than six hours of interviews, I wonder, how much jeopardy is their marriage in now? What has been lost more than gained by this husband and wife, married nearly 17 years, and missed by their daughters from not having had a home of their own for as long as their girls can remember? These are the questions Michelle is asking of herself, too.

Michelle hears LeRoy and his sister talking as if their mother will return to the apartment at home when discharged from the hip surgery rehabilitation. "But his mother can't get in and out of bed on her own," Michelle says, exasperated by the thought. "She is paranoid, hears terrifying voices, and is in and out of reality. I was wearing a hat the last time I saw her in the rehab center, and she said, 'How did you get here? Did your mommy drop you off?' She thought I was 13-year-old Katrina." Michelle knows that her mother-in-law needs round-the-clock care at home, but that's more than the family can afford.

Michelle hopes that LeRoy was listening as "his closest friend at work was talking about having just lost his mother. He told LeRoy that he and his brothers' decision to put their mother, who had dementia, in a nursing home two or three years ago was the best thing they could have done for her and for the whole family."

Recently Michelle asked LeRoy, "Have you asked our girls how they feel about this?"

"What Katrina said to me," Michelle told LeRoy, "is that she didn't want Grandma here anymore, but that she feels really bad saying that. Another time, Katrina asked, 'Why is our grandmother still with us?'"

What Michelle wants to say to LeRoy is that "it's okay not to see your mother every day." She also is planning to say to her husband, "We need to sit down and think about what is best for our family—and not just what might be best for your mother. *I can't take this anymore!*"

Has LeRoy so long been yielding to the family members who barked the loudest and demanded the most of him, however unreasonable his mother's and sister's expectations were and are? "It's time for LeRoy to let go," Michelle says, close to drawing a line in the sand. "He's still trying to hold on. What is it? A promise he made long ago to his mother? He has given her 61 years of his life. What about *us*?"

Michelle is planning ahead for a heart-to-heart conversation with LeRoy this weekend. She will ask him a couple of days earlier to save Saturday morning so he will know an important conversation lies ahead. Michelle will get coffee and bagels and they'll go his office where, on a Saturday, they can be alone. She is a wise young woman who loves her husband and can trust her own good heart to express in a loving way the serious and utterly reasonable concerns she has for the welfare of their marriage and family. Michelle will use her own hard-won insights and judgment to guide her and enlist LeRoy to work with her toward what the two of them can decide is best for their family.

LeRoy and Michelle love each other and their girls so much that focusing together on protecting these precious relationships may be how they share any final decisions. A "line in the sand" drawn by either of them won't work because Michelle or LeRoy could always blame their life partner for a decision forced upon the other one.

Whether Michelle's mother-in-law goes into a nursing home or back to the big house is a decision they have to make *together*. This is neither his sister's decision nor a choice to be made by anyone other than LeRoy and his wife, except with consideration for the welfare of Katrina and Kalya. If the couple can't yet come to an agreement, they will need to find a temporary place where LeRoy's mother can receive care. For the love of each other and their future as a family, they may need a marriage and family counselor's help to come to a loving and mutually chosen decision.

A FINAL THOUGHT

For caregivers who find themselves in difficult situations that seem beyond their power to resolve, professional guidance can offer a lifeline. The decision to place a loved one in a facility is not easy. This much is clear: Michelle and LeRoy are at a painful decision point, and, whatever decision they make as a couple, it will not put an end to all their concerns. As Cindy's experience in looking after her mother and her sister shows, the challenges of caregiving never stopped as long as they lived, but today, now that both are gone, the rewards remain to comfort Cindy and guide her in planning for her own and her husband's later years.

9

Truly Helpful Caregiving Tips

It isn't Alzheimer's [or another frailty] that takes away the person's dignity; it's other people's reactions that do.
—Joanne Koenig Coste, *Learning to Speak Alzheimer's*

A small suggestion, new insight, or problem-solving strategy can make a huge difference in reducing your caregiver stress and making your loved one more comfortable. Many of the experts I've studied and the scores of caregivers I've interviewed offer tips they've tried. Wrapped up in the tips they shared are empowering perspectives, practical solutions, and helpful ways of responding to common behaviors and concerns. As you read this chapter, I hope you will have many more than a few "ah-ha!" moments. Often the best ideas are like the proverbial elephant in a room: as soon as we become aware of what is obvious, we wonder why we never saw it before.

WHEN YOUR FAMILY MEMBER
OR FRIEND IS NEWLY DIAGNOSED

In her article in the *Washington Post*, Susan Berger tells of crossing paths with a longtime friend. She "looked great and was her typically upbeat, energetic self," but the woman shocked the journalist by announcing that she'd been recently diagnosed with early-stage Alzheimer's. "I hugged her and told her how sorry I was," Berger recalled. "Told her there are no words. In a daze, I finished my shopping. Driving home, I burst into tears." Many months later, Berger saw her friend at a distance at their local synagogue. Not knowing if she'd still be recognized or what to say, she remembers feeling relieved they weren't close enough to speak.

150

But later, her friend, now 73, was happy to tell Berger how she wants the world to relate to her: "She said she has a core group of girlfriends who treat her as before—including her in their plans for lunches, dinners, and outings to art galleries and museums," Berger explains. Her husband helps her do what she loves to do, from baking to putting on makeup, and lifts her spirits when she feels down. When she worries aloud what the Alzheimer's will do to her next, he tells her, "We don't know what is next. And we are all going to die someday. Let's just make this a good day."[1]

When a debilitating illness is moving in like an approaching hurricane, it's important to continue pleasurable activities as long as possible. Berger quotes Ruth Drew, a director at the Alzheimer's Association, who describes a man, once a very good golfer, now losing his ability to play: "But he didn't care," because he got out on the course with a volunteer from Drew's organization. "They drove around in a golf cart on a beautiful day and had a wonderful time. The outings were so meaningful. They made him feel regular—that he could still enjoy the things he enjoyed."[2]

Experts, Berger writes, suggest taking cues from the person with Alzheimer's. "If a newly diagnosed friend looks confused after you say hello, immediately say your name and mention how you know one another. ('Our kids went to school together.') But these reminders shouldn't feel like a test or a quiz. (Don't say: 'Remember? Our kids went to school together.') Tell the person, 'It's wonderful to see you.'"[3]

I recommend that you also tell friends and family members, "Please come visit. Mother loves having company and seeing familiar faces. She has good days and bad days. Sometimes her memory works rather well and sometimes not, but she gets lonely when no one comes to share lunch or take her out for a drive."

Affirm Dignity and Avoid "Excess Disability"

Joanne Koenig Coste, in *Learning to Speak Alzheimer's*, tells the story of a mother whose daughter no longer allows her to do the laundry. "She says it makes more work for her when I do it," the mother complains. "She says I forget the detergent. Imagine that. 'Don't go near the wash while I'm out, Mama,' she says to me, as if I'm a child."[4]

Her daughter could help her maintain her dignity by taking some simple steps that Coste suggests. For example, the daughter could place the detergent with a simple list of instructions by the washing machine, use bright nail polish to mark the usual settings on the washer and dryer, and follow the same day and time schedule for doing the laundry once a week. When that becomes no longer possible, the daughter could ask her mother to fold the clean laundry, "a repetitive task that [she] could still accomplish." If the daughter would then thank her for helping out, both of them could feel good.[5]

Helping your elderly impaired loved one feel useful is essential, explains Coste. "Even for people with Alzheimer's, life is about doing and not just being. 'What can I do—to help, to serve, to feel like a contributing part of family and community' is the silent plea of people with progressive dementia." The day program my friend Marian's mom attended had the attendees refold laundry many times after quickly running the towels through the dryer so they were warm. The staff was careful not to be obvious about it.

CREATIVE INTERVENTIONS FOR HANDLING HALLUCINATIONS, IMAGININGS, AND PARANOIA

Sometimes in disability or old age, we need to sleep with a light on, not only to be able to find the bathroom without falling over something but because of "sundowning." This disorientation or distortion of reality typically occurs later in the day and is experienced by 20 to 40 percent of people with dementia. In some ways these misperceptions are akin to the nighttime anxieties that many children experience.

When my daughter Ashley was little, she went through a period of being afraid of ghosts when it was dark. After several nights of being awakened and called to her bedroom, I asked her where the ghosts were. When she pointed to the closet, I headed there, loudly saying, "Alright, get out of here, you ghosts! I'm tired of you bothering my little girl!" Stomping my feet all the way, I marched the "ghosts" from her bedroom and out the front door, yelling, "Get out of here! And don't ever come back!" When I returned to Ashley's bedside, I brushed my hands back and forth together in the air, as if clanging cymbals, and declared, "They're gone!" Not saying a word, Ashley looked at me with the sweetest little wry smile and a face that bespoke triumph. In that moment, I was her all-powerful mommy. We had both triumphed—and the "ghosts" never came back.

Who? What? Where? When? How?

Author Laura Wayman was the manager of a home care company when an emergency call came from a worried niece who lived several hours away from her Aunt Edna. The distressed elderly aunt living alone in a big house, not far from Wayman's agency, had phoned her niece because there were "clowns" in her house. The week before, Aunt Edna had called 911 for help getting the clowns out, but the police left after saying that there were none. "They left me alone with them," Edna told Wayman.

In *A Loving Approach to Dementia Care*, Wayman describes the "creative intervention" she used that brought comfort and calm to Aunt Edna. Responding in a way often effective in tamping down the anxiety that flows from irrational, distorted fears of things seen or unseen, the first thing that Wayman did was to listen to Edna's fears. She did not try to dismiss them. Instead, she asked open-ended questions. "Where are the clowns now?" Aunt Edna pointed to where they sat and told Wayman they came for the clothes they said she had taken from them. "Where are the clothes?" Edna led Wayman to her bedroom closet and pulled out the items she said the clowns wanted. As Wayman took the clothes to her car, she recalls, "I looked over my shoulder and said to the nonexistent clowns, 'This is all of it. I will take the clothes and you back to where you belong, and you must never come here again and bother this nice lady.'"[6]

Accepting Edna's answers to her reality, Wayman explains, was key to tracking down the specifics and solving the problem. When a cognitively impaired person is having hallucinations or making accusations of stealing, not reacting but "coping with and managing [such behaviors] is the key to making the person feel safe and supported."[7]

In his 80s and 90s, my dad didn't have memory problems, but he did have episodes of paranoia. Daddy would get the idea that one or another of us children was maliciously doing something against him, and for days or weeks at a time he would feel "wronged." Sometimes he stayed focused on these suspicious ideas the way his old birddog, Daisy, used to stand motionless, again and again, her eyes riveted on another bevy of quail. Once Daddy surprised me by claiming, "Your brother wants to be king! He's planning to sell the farmland and keep all the money for himself!"

Dumbfounded, I said, "Oh, that's not true," and no more. Our dad was an old-fashioned disciplinarian. We didn't have much practice in speaking up for ourselves, even as adults. I *wanted* to say, "Daddy, Vaughn is a loyal son! He comes often, from all the way across the country, to help you and Mama." I *wanted* to remind him that my brother was a highly successful engineer. Not only was my brother an honorable man, he didn't need or want the family's wheat fields. But I couldn't say so to my father. He and my mother had worked hard to leave us the farmland both of their parents had passed down to them. Using logic would not have lessened my father's paranoid ideas, just intensified his resentments.

I wish I had known when my parents were in their late life years what I have learned from Laura Wayman: Whether your loved one has dementia or is just cantankerous and difficult in other ways, the best way to approach irrational, suspicious thinking is simply to listen and ask open-ended questions. Sometimes changing the subject or distracting a person by getting him or her to talk about meaningful life experiences or playing familiar music is an effective way to respond. But the who? what? where? when? how? approach is a far more effective way to calm down a fearful person making accusations. When my father got it in his head that one of us siblings was doing something against him, I should have asked, "Who said this?" or, "What makes you think that's going on?" or "Where did this happen?" or, "When did you start feeling this way?" and, "How could that happen?"

YES, THERE *CAN* BE TOO MUCH OF A GOOD THING

Like the "Tiger Mom" who devotes her energy and fervent attention to giving her child every possible opportunity, some care providers are *overly conscientious*. Perhaps the person who tries "too hard" to care for their impaired loved one might best be described as a "Tiger Caregiver." Might this be a description of you?

By trying to do all the right things, you may inadvertently be putting the person you care for in a straitjacket, resulting in a struggle you don't want. You will want to avoid creating a situation where the proverbial perfect becomes the enemy of the good. Just as a child needs recess during the school day, your loved one needs to "catch a break" from doing what you've decided is "good for her" or "in his best interest." Whatever our age, none of us wants to be *constrained or forced* to behave in certain ways. It should come as no surprise that elders with neurocognitive disabilities become agitated, aggressive, uncooperative, or tearful when coerced into doing something they don't want to do.

Sometimes, for example, an argument erupts over taking pills. You may think you're not a good caregiver if you don't give the medicines exactly as directed on the prescription's label. But maybe there isn't a fixed timetable. Why not ask the doctor, "How much leeway do I have? Are there certain medicines that have to be given exactly as specified?" You may learn there is some "wiggle room" that allows you to say, "Okay. We can wait awhile on these pills." It may not matter if it's before breakfast or after, at three o'clock or four. By not insisting on a rigid timetable on a day when he or she just doesn't want to do it, you may be able to avoid creating a "meltdown situation" that is distressing for you both.

"*A person's feelings also affect his behavior,*" emphasize the authors of *The 36-Hour Day*, the bible of family guidebooks on dementia care. Nancy Mace and Peter Rabins give a powerful description of the importance of empathy and a problem-solving approach:

> The person who has dementia probably feels lost, worried, anxious, vulnerable, and helpless much of the time. He may also be aware that he fails at tasks and feel that he is making a fool of himself. Imagine what he must feel like if he wants to say something nice to his caregiver but all that comes out are curse words. Think how frightening it must be if a familiar home and familiar people now seem strange and unfamiliar. If we can find ways to make the person who has dementia feel more secure and comfortable, behavioral symptoms may decline.[8]

AVOIDING THE "CATASTROPHIC" SITUATION

When experience tells you the behavior you are seeing is the prelude to an emotional overreaction, you can prevent the crisis by backing off: "Well, we don't have to do that right now. Tell me what *you'd* like to do. What would you enjoy?" Does it really matter if she has her bath right now? Will the world end if he wears the same trousers he wore yesterday and the day before? Does he really have to go to that doctor if she's going to make him feel like a fool by asking him to do all those things he can't do anymore, like draw a clock or count backwards? If there's no good reason to insist on keeping that appointment, you can cancel it or go there together and say to your dad's physician, "He doesn't want to do those memory questions. It just makes him feel sad."

No Adult Wants to Be Treated Like a Child

In every stage of life, our yearning for more self-determination deserves to be acknowledged. As parents we may assume that a young child is "just being a spoiled brat" when the child, who may be expressing genuine distress, "throws a fit" and refuses to do something we ask. Scolding the child makes it more likely that the child's tantrum will continue, while ignoring it more readily calms things down. Similarly, caregivers often label impaired elderly persons as "stubborn" when their behavior may be a normal reaction to a frustrating situation. No one likes to be bossed around, and no adult wants to be treated like a child. By focusing more on the quality of your relationship than whatever task is at hand—showing your elderly loved one deference and respect—you may prevent many catastrophic situations from happening.

Elders need to do what they can still do for themselves, emphasizes Keren Brown Wilson, the woman who pioneered "methods of compassionate care" that became the Oregon model of assisted living, replicated widely in the United States and in countries in Latin America. She emphasizes that helping vulnerable elders *live* is no easy task. "Dressing somebody is easier than letting them dress themselves. It takes less time. It's less aggravation."[9]

In assisted living facilities and nursing homes, writes physician Atul Gawande in *Being Mortal: Medicine and What Matters in the End*, "unless supporting people's capabilities is made a priority, the staff ends up dressing people like they are rag dolls. Gradually, that's how everything begins to go. The tasks come to matter more than the people."[10]

Try not to undertake time-consuming activities, such as getting your loved one bathed or dressed to go someplace, when you or your paid caregivers are overly tired, preoccupied with other concerns, or pressed for time. By slowing down some caregiving tasks to give yourself and your loved one more time, rather than rushing, you may be able to avoid triggering a catastrophic reaction that results in crying, screaming, or lashing out on the care recipient's part and frustration on the caregiver's part.

Tiring and time-consuming caregiving activities are more successfully accomplished during the "best times of the day"—when your loved one tends to be in a better mood and both of you are better able to handle stress. An impaired person functions best in a peaceful environment with less noise and when your demeanor is warm and engaging.

A well-organized approach to caregiving can make all the difference, too. In *Learning to Speak Alzheimer's*, Joanne Koenig Coste provides a number of valuable tips on helping patients dress. She advises selecting clothes that are familiar and recognizable to the patient, as well as comfortable and easy to put on and take off. For example, she suggests looking for loose-fitting shirts and dresses that slip on over the head, pants that have elastic waists, and slip-on shoes. Avoid zippers and try buying clothes that are one size larger than usual.[11]

Coste also suggests keeping a "behavior log" to identify what triggers challenging behavior. A pattern will emerge within 10 journal entries, she says, if you record "the time of the day, the exact location of the behavior, and a thorough description of the environmental elements such as odors, sights, and sounds." Once you know the time slot and circumstances of the triggering events, you can change whatever needs changing:[12] for example, turn off the TV, make the room warmer or cooler, have the grandkids move their play farther away, or find something pleasurable for him or her to do (help set the dinner table or go on a walk with a family member).

Researchers Claudia Miranda-Castillo, Bob Woods, and Martin Orrell tell us that "when people with dementia are involved in their care and have felt a part of the decision-making process, there has been an improvement in their quality of life." Involving your loved one in decisions about their day-to-day activities also has been shown to raise their self-esteem.[13]

To the greatest extent possible, given your loved one's condition, offer him or her choices, but not too many at once: "Shall we buy these blue slacks or the green ones?" or, "Would you like the TV on or off? Is this program okay or do you want to watch something else?" or, "How about some oatmeal for breakfast today, or would you prefer scrambled eggs?" or, "Do you want to see the doctor about that pain in your hip?"

Help from Mother Nature—and Your Own Wise Responses

For many elderly people, "sleep-wake disturbances, sundowning, and other time disorientations" are common occurrences, because their internal time clocks are disturbed, writes John Zeisel in *I'm Still Here: A New Philosophy of Alzheimer's Care*. For them, physical contact with nature can be helpful by tying them to "the time of day, the weather, and the passing of the seasons [so] people living with Alzheimer's remain aware of time passing," Zeisel explains, having observed the related positive effects of gardens, porches, and patios.[14] Experts also recommend an hour of sunshine in the morning, exercise and other stimulating afternoon activities, night-lights, and regular bedtimes to improve the quality and peacefulness of nighttime sleep.[15]

Repeatedly reminding a cognitively impaired person where he or she is, and always explaining what is going on, can ease the task of coping with the stress of memory problems and misperceptions. It's hard not to take it personally if your mother mistakes you for your sister, forgets who your children are, or if your husband asks, "Who are you?" Tell yourself, *"This is the disease of dementia speaking,"—not the person you love.* The best way to respond is to answer, "It's me, Mom. I'm Ann. Let me show you some wonderful photos of your grand-daughters." Or, "I'm your wife, Angela. I live here with you. I love you and I take good care of you."

When I would visit my own mother in her last years, six or eight times a day I showed her photographs of my daughters as babies, little and big girls, and college students—often with her in the picture, with me alongside. "This is Amanda. She's in college in Indiana. And this is Ashley. She goes to college at the University of Maryland," I would say, again and again. Mama said the exact same words every time: "Oh, they're so pretty! And you can tell they're smart, too!" I never got tired of hearing Mama say those sweet words! Rather than thinking it sad that her Alzheimer's disease was progressing, I thought it a blessing that my mother's good heart and exuberant pride in my daughters never wavered.

Psychologists Rose Oliver and Frances Bock, in *Coping with Alzheimer's: A Caregiver's Emotional Survival Guide*, give good advice on how to handle "difficult moments." First, don't take things personally. Even if your mother claims you've "stolen her new blouse," don't be hurt and don't get angry. Just say, "'Let's look in your closet together. We'll probably find it.' When you find it—as you probably will—say, 'Isn't it lucky that we found your blouse?'" If you can't find it, say, "'We'll look for it again after we've had our lunch.' A scene has been averted. She'll appreciate a hug."[16]

How We Frame a Stressful Situation Shapes Our Response

The way we look at problems determines our feelings. As Oliver and Bock explain, a person with dementia is not a spoiled child and should not be viewed as one. "Your husband is not in the same situation as a child who has not yet learned the limits of acceptable social behavior . . . Your husband is in the process of losing his ability to understand the world or what is expected of him in everyday situations . . . When he acts stubbornly, he is, in a way, saying, 'I am not a child. Don't treat me like one. I am still an autonomous person, and you can't make me do what I don't want to do.'"[17]

Of course, you can get angry, and who would blame you? But you'll probably feel better and handle the stress better if you decide not to and instead say to yourself, "He is acting dementedly, not childishly. That is the only way he knows how to act."[18]

"Fiblets" and Other Acts of Kindness

Sometimes total honesty is counterproductive, even cruel. Oliver and Bock suggest a different approach, using "creative evasions; half-truths that give comfort; reassurance instead of criticism; diversion instead of clashes of will." Respond to your loved one with empathy and kindness, not logic.[19] As gerontology experts Susan McCurry and Claudia Drossel explain, even if you are asked to hear the same story time after time, "What is to be gained by saying, 'Dad, you already told me that one'?"[20]

McCurry and Drossel go on to suggest that "compassionate misinformation" can shield the care recipient from painful realities. If a woman with dementia insists on saying that her son who died years ago will be arriving on a visit, don't correct her. Instead, ask her to share with you her memories of him. "Such reminiscences help the person with dementia connect their increasingly fragmented past and present, practice telling stories, and connect with another human being, even if the shared memories were never actual events."[21]

Compassionate misinformation can help families ease an elderly person with dementia into respite care or residential placement. Telling your impaired loved one "this move is for your own good" almost never works. What *can* make all the difference is using what you know about your loved one's personal history to meaningfully describe the changes ahead. McCurry and Drossel tell the story of Genevieve, who had lived with her husband in a condominium early in their marriage of more than 60 years. After he died, her family told her "that her husband had left her a condominium to care for her after his death, [and] she gladly moved to the room of the specialized dementia care unit. Once there, she continued to tell the staff how much her husband loved her and how he had bought the 'condo' for her."[22]

By managing your own behavior (not criticizing or raising your voice, staying calm, and remaining patient), you can set the tone for how your elderly loved one reacts. It is important to "pick your battles" and not to "correct or admonish unless the person is doing something unsafe or unhealthy."[23] Because keeping your emotions in check in highly stressful situations (and finding the right words) is so difficult to do, I've culled some helpful tips from a number of experts in the field.

"Ask Yourself: Would I Want to Be Talked to in This Way?"

McCurry and Drossel emphasize the importance of communicating respect, speaking in a way that isn't patronizing, and not lecturing.[24] They advise family members and professional care providers to offer individuals with dementia the opportunity to have conversations. Speak slowly to fit the abilities of the person, using short sentences. Smile and make eye contact, stand or sit at eye level, and speak only as loudly as necessary to make these conversations mutually enjoyable.[25]

Many paid caregivers, random strangers, and even medical professionals routinely call elderly people by their given names or casually say, "Dearie," "Sweetie," "Honey," or "Young Lady." In a recent *Huffington Post* article, "The Cruelty of Calling Older Adults 'Sweetie' or 'Honey,'" Debbie Reslock writes, "When asked, almost everyone agrees this behavior isn't intended to hurt anyone. But that doesn't take away the sting when it happens. Or the insult when a doctor talks to someone else about a patient, without permission or necessity, while that person is present. Not unlike the way he or she would do to a parent of a small child."[26]

As a simple matter of showing respect, everyone deserves to be addressed as they prefer: Mr., Mrs., Ms., Dr., Reverend, or "Miss Mary," by paid caregivers and nursing home staff, or George, Margaret, Aunt Lucy, or Grandpa by family. You can introduce your loved one to others accordingly, speak quietly, or slip a note to the person saying, "Please don't call my mom 'Young Lady,'" or, "Please call my dad Mr. Jones," or "Most people call my mom Dr. Smith." It is an indignity enough to be a physically or cognitively impaired adult, dependent on others for your care without having a young nursing aide or a doctor (who could be your son or granddaughter) call you by your first name.

An Adult Is Still an Adult in Old Age

Continuing her discussion of ageism, Reslock recalls the embarrassment on the face of a 91-year-old friend who was given "a bib to wear for dinner one night at his Denver nursing home. He usually ate alone in his room, but I'd stopped by for a late afternoon visit and he'd asked me to join him." He was a man she had long admired: "Besides being funny and incredibly kind, he was one of the wisest men I'd ever known. He also was a piano man in the Big Band era and had played with Glenn Miller. But that day, he was humiliated at being treated like a child in front of his friend."[27]

"Offer Praise When It Is Sincere"

Everyone appreciates encouraging words. When spoken to your elderly loved one in an adult-to-adult voice, not in a sing-song manner, as if you're praising a child, genuine compliments are a good thing. Treat your loved one as you hope to be treated when it's your turn to be old and vulnerable, with words of praise that communicate respect and warmth. As often as it is authentic, offer your support by saying, "Good job!"[28]

"Feeling Overwhelmed Isn't Surprising, Being Surprised about It Is"

In *Meditations for Women Who Do Too Much*, Anne Wilson Schaef observes that we, as caregivers—male or female—may feel overwhelmed because we expect too much of ourselves.[29] Thinking that only we can handle a situation and considering ourselves indispensable puts us on a path to a place "where we feel like saying 'to hell with everything.'" This is a sure signal that "we have not been taking care of ourselves."[30]

Writes Jolene Brackey, in *Creating Moments of Joy for the Person with Alzheimer's or Dementia*, "You better believe it—your mood does affect their mood! If you are rushed, they are rushed. If you're upset, they are upset. If you're happy, they are happy. Basically, you decide what kind of a day it's going to be. I am not saying it's easy. We all have bad days—that's life! Know that you can have bad days. You are human, not perfect." Brackey recommends that caregivers at home get started on the right foot by asking a family member or paid caregiver to bathe and dress your loved one each morning. Find a way to get an hour for yourself first, "and then the two of you can start your day together, refreshed and ready to go."[31]

You and your loved one both run an increased risk of suffering from depression if your needs for daytime activities and companionship aren't met.[32] Activities at home, designed to engage the individual being cared for, can reduce both behavioral symptoms and caregiver burden.[33] The quality of *your* life (reduced feelings of burden and increased sense of well being) and the quality of your loved one's life (social stimulation, meaningful leisure activities, and reduced psychological distress) almost surely will improve if you access the programs at your local senior center or utilize adult day care services. The Department of Aging in your area and Alzheimer's Association can refer you to the available community resources.

"When We Take Care of Ourselves, We Quit before We Are Forced to Our Knees"

You're not a bad person if you're exhausted, can't do this alone anymore, or just need a life of your own. Community-based services can offer information, emotional support, and respite care. An effective problem-focused approach to the challenges of elder care means *taking care of yourself and getting whatever help is needed* to solve the specific problems you're dealing with, one at a time.[34]

A six-year study by JoAnn Tschanz and her colleagues at Utah State University and the Johns Hopkins University School of Medicine found that when caregivers regularly used problem-solving strategies, patients with dementia showed slower rates of cognitive and functional decline.[35] If you see your loved one suddenly becoming agitated, for example, often you can resolve the problem by changing the environmental factor that triggers it. This practical approach offers several significant bonuses. For starters, setting aside your emotional response to the situation and focusing on solving the problem will give both you and your loved one more ability to cope. What's more, solving problems as they arise may slow down the progression of your loved one's illness. At the end of the day, using a problem-focused approach can help you experience more meaning in your role as caregiver and renew your resources as you continue to meet the challenges that lie ahead.[36]

How to Treat Yourself More Kindly

Once again, Oliver and Bock offer good advice: "Begin to appreciate yourself. Begin to give yourself positive messages. Begin to tell yourself, 'Even if he didn't appreciate the walk we took, or the new sweater I brought him, or the lunch I prepared, I feel good about doing these things because it was right and because I know that I'm doing the best that I can.' Learning to praise yourself for your own positive deeds will free you from the often futile search for praise from others."[37]

When things *don't* go well, when either you or your loved one, or both of you, have an awful day, remind yourself that tomorrow is another day. "You get to start over fresh," adds Brackey. "The person with dementia doesn't remember what happened yesterday."[38]

And, finally, from Pauline Boss, author of *Loving Someone Who Has Dementia: How to Find Hope While Coping with Stress and Grief*, comes this advice: "Don't aim for perfection. Just do the best you can. If you feel as though it's never enough, know that this feeling is typical for most caregivers. Make your peace . . . you still have the power to accept what there is as good enough. That part is within your control."[39]

When Your Loved One Dies—
Relief, Grief, and Moving Forward

> You should think of this period of time immediately following your [loved
> one's] death as a time of transition, a time to explore a direction that
> is right for you . . . Allowing yourself a time of transition and labeling it
> as such is a good idea. You need time to grieve and renew yourself.
> —Clinical social workers Esther Lebow and Barbara Kane,
> *Coping with Your Difficult Older Parent*

In this chapter, I will share the individual stories of a daughter, a wife, and a
husband—as each of them freely gave years of support and caregiving to their
loved one—each of whom, after their loved one's death, experienced relief,
grief, and renewal. Each story is as different as were the caregivers and those
they cared for. Yet some common themes run through them all. There is the
initial inability to grasp the seriousness of the loved one's condition and prognosis followed by the ongoing and ever-changing challenges of finding the
help they and their loved ones needed. Caregivers struggled, whether it was
just to get through the day, find medical treatment, or deal with family issues.
They grieved even as they coped and saw to their loved ones' needs.

The first story, of Joyce and her mom, relates the guilt that caregivers feel
when the answer is nursing home placement. The stories that follow delve into
the difficulties of caring for a spouse through decline and death. One story
relates caring for a once-vibrant man changed by illness into someone almost
unrecognizable. Another tells of a wife and mother dying while her youngest
child is still at home.

Each story gives a look into the challenges the caregivers faced and how they met them. I owe a debt of thanks to all the caregivers, in this chapter and throughout this book, who shared their stories with me—stories that bring valuable caregiving and healing lessons. These survivors tell us that, even after great grief, it is possible to once again experience joy, find new meaning, and cherish new connections in life.

And now, their stories.

JOYCE AND HER MOM

Did there ever come a time when I prayed that my mother would die? Absolutely! I thought she had no quality of life whatsoever. I didn't feel sad when she died, and for several weeks after. I felt such relief that her suffering was over. Maybe a month later, I wondered, "Why did it have to end this way?" I was grieving, feeling pretty depressed. I kept thinking, "Oh, God, this is terrible! It was such a terrible way to die." My mother didn't deserve that!

—Joyce

Mrs. Taylor, Joyce's mother, was almost 86 when she died, just about a year ago. She was a resilient person, and for the first few of her seven years as a widow, Mrs. Taylor's family helped her live a mostly enjoyable life. "Mom was always at my house for holidays, family birthdays, and once a week to have lunch, get her hair done, and have dinner," Joyce recalls. "Her apartment was in a four-story building for low-income seniors, and the four of us sibs (my sisters Phyllis and Donna, brother Earl, and me) took turns visiting her on weekends. We'd take her out to eat or bring her a meal. When she could no longer drive and had memory problems, she needed our visits more often."

Joyce remembers that, "for a long time, I was in denial over just how impaired my mother was becoming. She had always been so strong." With five children, and barely scraping by on the family's modest income, Joyce's mother had been a loving caregiver to Joyce's severely disabled kid sister until she died at the age of eighteen. "I admired my mother and saw her as always able to do whatever was needed."

On the days when Joyce came to take her mother home for the day, she would have her baby grandson in the back seat, and would call her mother ahead of time, to come downstairs and be there when Joyce arrived to pick her up. "When I arrived," Joyce went on, "sometimes she'd still be in her pajamas in her apartment because she had forgotten all about my phone call minutes earlier. We'd get home and I would set her up downstairs, in a chair with a table, where she could eat lunch. If I was working in the kitchen and had left the room, I'd come back and she wouldn't have eaten anything. I had to say, 'Mom, eat your lunch.' Then she'd focus her attention and remember to eat."

Continuing to be surprised by her mother's increasingly steep cognitive decline, Joyce said, "My mother was always a neat freak, but I noticed she wasn't doing any cleaning anymore. She never in a million years would not have made her bed. So when I arrived one morning and saw her lying on top of the bedspread, it took me a minute to realize that she'd never changed out of her clothes from the night before."

Finding Available Help

Joyce started checking on her mother more often and signed her up for the evening meal that was provided at a low cost in the dining room downstairs, but her mom would forget to go. "One of the days when I came straight from work to take her down to dinner, my mother fell while I was there. Because I had to go somewhere, this nice woman named Esther, who was one of the younger residents, volunteered to make sure my mother got safely back to her apartment. After that, I approached Esther and asked if she could walk Mom back every evening, after I took her down and stayed with her at dinner for 40 or 45 minutes." That worked well, but it soon became clear that more help was needed.

"The person who ran the front desk," Joyce told me, "knew everybody's business in the whole building, and offered us some advice. Someone who didn't live in the building was coming to visit another resident, and maybe she could also visit our mom every day. We paid this woman $14 or $15 an hour to come at lunchtime to be sure our mother ate. Then I asked her to come in the mornings, too, to make sure Mom took her medicine."

Joyce told the hired helper, "Whatever food is in Mom's apartment for you to make her for breakfast, we'd like you to fix the same for yourself and eat with her." The arrangement worked well to provide care for Joyce's mother, several days a week for a number of months. In addition, the family paid Esther to keep coming on some days, for a few more hours of companionship and support.

When Assisted Living Is Anything but That

"One day Esther found my mother on the floor when she arrived in the morning. We had to move Mom into assisted living. It was a place not far from where I live. There were 15 elderly residents there, with two caregivers working 12-hour shifts."

Joyce and her siblings felt guilty that the family couldn't find or afford something better. More paid caregivers were needed to help their mother and the other residents do things for themselves and stay mobile as long as possible. "If I had been a wealthy person," Joyce lamented, "my mother would have been at my house, and I'd have hired help that I could watch to be sure that she got good care."

Her mother went to the facility able to walk to the bathroom on her own, with a walker. "Later we realized that, for their convenience," Joyce continued, "the staff had been putting Mom in a wheelchair to go to the toilet rather than taking the time to let her walk. Before long, my mother lost her strength and could hardly walk."

In his best-selling book *Being Mortal*, physician Atul Gawande notes that finding an assisted living place that actually *helps people with living* is easier said than done. What staff members often care most about is saving time and making things easier for themselves.[1] Instead of supporting people so they can function as long as possible, putting elders unnecessarily in wheelchairs increases their dependency and further robs them of dignity.

"If You Don't Have a Boatload of Money"

"We tried to solve problems as best we could, to take care of our mother. But if you don't have a boatload of money, some things are out of your control," Joyce explained. "We knew that a more expensive facility wouldn't necessarily give our mother better care, but more paid caregivers were needed, and that just wasn't affordable." Their mother's Social Security wasn't enough income. Joyce and her siblings had to use her savings to pay a couple thousand dollars a month for basic care. "We were blessed in our family because Mom did not give us a fit. Mom never said, 'When am I going home?' She seemed fine with assisted living and stayed there for almost two years."

Joyce was "still in denial," she told me. "If I was in the driver's seat, Mom probably would have stayed in assisted living longer." It was her sister, Phyllis, a nurse and the one who always took their mom to her doctor's appointments, who saw with clarity that their mother's condition now required a nursing home. "Mom's condition was getting so bad, she just had to be moved somewhere that was not so understaffed. My sister Phyllis took care of all the hard stuff including applying for the Medicaid approval that took forever to come through for Mom, which seemed to be the norm."

At the nursing home, "Some of the patients were still able to enjoy the man who came in with a keyboard once a week to play old familiar songs, or attend religious services, and other occasional events. But my mother was pretty much unable to find pleasure in those kinds of things by the time she began to live there." When Joyce came to visit, her mother would usually be in a wheelchair in the dining room, Joyce explained. "I would take her back to her room where it was quiet. There was a TV in there, and I'd stay while she had her dinner. The other nursing home patients looked like they were falling out of their chairs, so I'd always get something to put under Mom's arms to prop her up, so she could at least be comfortable and stay upright."

"At the Nursing Home They Acted Like They Cared More Than They Did"

It bothered Joyce that "there was so much pretense. The aides working there at the nursing home, when a patient had a visitor, would be calling everyone 'Sweetheart' and 'Honey,' and they treated the patient a whole lot nicer. I totally get it that patients can be hard to take care of, and if I'd have been working there 8–10 hours and was getting such low pay, I might have yelled at somebody, too. But it still bothered me that the nursing aides often acted like they cared more than they did."

When Joyce would see another patient who needed help, she'd tell one of the aides about it, but the aide would reply, "She's not *my* patient." It troubled Joyce that, "while some of the nursing aides were good, others when you called attention to a problem, they always had an excuse for not addressing it."

On the days of the week when she wasn't driving more than two hours in heavy traffic to spend a few days helping her daughter with baby twins, Joyce was working a part-time job, then going straight to the nursing home after work. With a husband and another grandchild locally who had two working parents, there was a lot of fatigue and stress to cope with. Even so, Joyce and her sisters tried to do nice things for the patients and staff, such as bringing in cookies or getting little gifts for the aides' birthdays. They also tried to compliment or thank their mother's caregivers at every opportunity.

"Both of my sisters did a better job than I did of speaking up for our mother's care, and making complaints when needed," Joyce said. "My sister Donna, who was having major health problems and was in a lot of pain, gave Mom a lot of quality time. Phyllis gave Mom manicures and was our mother's constant advocate for nursing care. When I was there, I would feed my mother and help the aide change my mother's diaper. Some of the other patients never had anyone visit, so we tried to be nice to them, too."

It upset Joyce when she walked in to see her mother lying in bed. Almost always there was dried food that had spilled and was stuck various places on her bedspread. Joyce kept bringing in clean blankets and taking the others home to wash. "Whenever I was there, I would feed her and I saw that, the way her room was set up, the aides would need to face my mother to feed her, with the TV at their backs. Mom's blanket was always so disgustingly layered with spilled food that I wondered if they just fed her while watching television, instead of facing her and treating her like a person.

"Last December, before she died in May," Joyce recalled, reexperiencing feelings of outrage and heartbreak, "I found a sore on Mom's foot, and she never got out of bed again until she died. I called Phyllis and said, 'Mom's got this disgusting bed sore on her foot! The nursing aide said Mom got it from the rubber air mattress that you brought her a couple days ago. I said to the nurse in charge, there's *no way* she got that sore in two days!'" Joyce knew that "whoever had been bathing my mother didn't take her socks off, or they'd have seen this terrible wound!"

Joyce proudly relates the fact that Phyllis went straightaway to the head nurse's supervisor. "We need a meeting," Phyllis said. "I'm not happy with my mother's care! This woman [the head nurse] does not make her employees do what they're supposed to do! She yells, 'Fire!' after it's too late. As a registered nurse, I worked in a nursing home, and you can't tell me anything!"

Soon after, they placed their mom in hospice care. Once hospice started, hospice workers left little books in their mother's room at the nursing home. The books told Joyce and her siblings about the progression of their mother's disease and what to expect as their mother was nearing the end of her life.

"Mom hadn't been eating, and the lady from the hospice told us, 'You're a week or two away from dying when you stop eating and drinking.' That

Sunday, when I got there after church, she was breathing really weird. I remembered hearing other people talk about a 'death rattle.' I went home to tell my husband, and not long after that, we were called and told to get right back there."

After her mom died two days later, Joyce's first response was relief. Many others I've counseled, comforted as friends, or interviewed for this book (and I, myself, on losing my granny) have felt the same. Recalling her mother's last several years with an ever-diminishing quality of life, unable to feed herself and bedridden for the last five months, Joyce said, "I just thanked God that her suffering was over. It is such an indignity to be like that."

Knowing that *her mother would not want to have been kept alive* in her deteriorated condition, Joyce could be at peace. She had cared for her mother the best she could and knew her mother (had her mind been capable of such reasoning) would be happy that Joyce's caregiving energies could now more freely focus on her newborn twin granddaughters and other grandchildren.

Looking Ahead to Her Own Old Age

Joyce's older daughter has four children, including babies who are twins, and the family lives in another state. "She will be parenting little kids for a long time," Joyce explained. "My younger daughter, who lives close by, has one child, and she is the one I worry about, when it comes to my getting old. I keep thinking about how hard it will be for Dawn. So my joke is, when we pass an assisted living place near her house, 'Oh, there's my future home!'

"In truth," Joyce continued, "I want to say to Dawn, I don't want you to do some of the things I did. I don't want you to have your whole holiday wrapped around me. The last time I brought Grandma home for Christmas Eve, she was still in assisted living. She didn't know anything except that it was raining a freezing rain, and she was mad about it. If I hadn't brought her to the house that day, it wouldn't have made any difference."

Remembering the troublesome feelings with which she was struggling, Joyce continued, "Sometimes, the things I did were guilt-driven. If I'm old and suffering with a poor quality of life, and if I need surgery and won't get better even if I have the surgery, I'm telling my daughters, '*Don't you decide* I should have that surgery.'"

Looking ahead, Joyce also wants to tell her daughters, "If Daddy and I are both alive and Daddy is taking care of *me* in an apartment, I want you to make sure you *get* him some help. Not *give* him help. Get adult day care for me. He won't want you to do it, but have someone in to help him."

Joyce feels a deep sense of relief. Throughout her mother's years of living with the progressively debilitating, ravaging illness of dementia, Joyce and her siblings provided their mom with the best life that they could give her, all things considered. Joyce is thankful that her mother is no longer suffering the undeserved indignities, one after another, that broke Joyce's heart to watch, especially as she recalled the extraordinary acts of love and care her mom gave her severely disabled sister for the 18 years that she lived.

These days, Joyce enjoys planning and taking vacations with her husband in his retirement. They enjoy being actively involved in the lives of five precious grandchildren. They share good times with friends. He keeps busy with handyman projects around the house, and she has more time for her church and community service activities. Joyce and her husband realize that the gifts of good health and meaningful lives—not to be taken for granted—are blessings to be cherished as long as possible.

JOANNE AND HER HUSBAND

Joanne and Walt, both marrying for the second time in 1974, were a perfect match in their mutual enjoyment of outdoor adventures and indoor experiences of the arts. Living in western Massachusetts, the couple loved snowmobiling, skiing, camping, and motorcycling. They took joy in all their adventures, from sleeping in a pup tent and drinking campfire coffee, to driving their motorcycles to Tanglewood, where they'd put their helmets aside and sit back to enjoy a concert.

Years of Joy

From the mid-70s through the 1980s, Walt was an information technology specialist and businessman. Joanne, by her own description, was a "college dropout" who worked her way up from marketing jobs at a bank and radio station to become a successful fund-raiser for public television. They bought a sailboat and named her *Joy*. Sailing together brought Joanne, Walt, his children, and their friends "tremendous fun" for more than 24 years. When he retired, Walt said, "Joanne, it's your turn. You have it in you to bloom like a rose." Her work took her abroad to book talent, and Walt accompanied her. He was proud of Joanne and bragged about her to others.

This "wonderfully spirited man who loved life showed me what it was to live," Joanne told me. "I'm definitely who I've become because of him."

"I Lost Him a Long Time before I Lost Him"

They were both longtime smokers, but Joanne quit in her mid-40s, after surviving a bout with cancer. Walt continued to smoke into his late 70s and was oxygen support dependent with emphysema for the last eight years of his life.

About the time Joanne retired, five years before Walt's death, he crashed into the back of a car sitting at a stoplight. He suffered a blunt chest trauma, his breathing problems significantly worsened, and Joanne's caregiving responsibilities escalated. They had been traveling back and forth from Massachusetts to their condominium in South Carolina, which now became their home for more months of the year.

Shortly after the auto accident, Walt fell and broke his hip. His hip surgery wasn't very successful. "That was the beginning of wheeling him around in a wheelchair," Joanne explained. "His knees were bone on bone and constantly hurting, and for the rest of his life he was taking pain medications." Joanne set up an Excel spreadsheet just to keep track of his medications, most of them opioids for pain.

He was not a man you could argue with. "Walt was taking 23 pills a day," Joanne recalls. "Those drugs became the most important thing in his life, and he was constantly swearing: 'Goddamn this. Goddamn that. Get me some goddamn tea, Joanne.' My ears were so violated every time he spoke.

"Faithful to my marriage vows—in sickness and in health—it was a hard journey," Joanne told me, tearfully. "Those last four or five years, he had no filter. He said whatever came to the top of his mind. My name was 'goddamnit, Joanne.' He'd see a pretty girl and say, 'She'd be great in the sack, she and her big boobs!'"

What was worse, "Walt seemed to take joy in making me squirm. If I would challenge him, his voice would rise and his words would be even more hurtful. After a while, I didn't want to hear him open his mouth."

Joanne realized then, "I lost him a long time before I lost him." When I asked how she coped with his verbal abuse and the stress that went on for nearly five years, Joanne said, "You can't dwell on it. Here's the situation. Make the best of it. You have to move on. In my family, we were raised to be stoic."

Having her brother and sister-in-law living in the condo next door to theirs in South Carolina helped Joanne find relief in daily, hour-long walks. "After Walt took his morning meds," she explained, "I would leave the door open, never locked, and my brother or his wife would look in to check on Walt. In addition to walking, about once a week I would play golf."

Finding Strength

What also helped to relieve Joanne's stress and provide regular respite was Walt's habit of wanting daily to be wheeled down to the condominium's swimming pool. "From about noon until six, with beer, ice tea, and Pepsi in a cooler on the back of his wheelchair," Joanne explained, Walt, with his oxygen canister, sat under an umbrella. Still a personable guy with most people, he visited with the residents who came to the community pool to swim or relax in nearby lounge chairs. "The pool boy would periodically take Walt to the bathroom. From our condo, I could look down to see that Walt was okay, sitting under that umbrella." Those six hours, in decent weather, on most days of the week, gave Joanne a chance to be alone, read a good book, or visit with friends. She also found strength from her faith and regularly attending Mass.

Walt was diagnosed with lung cancer two years before his death. There were many episodes of Walt desperately crying out, "Joanne, I can't breathe!" A number of times, he was rushed to a local emergency room. Walt got to the place of being so frail, hostile, miserable, and profane that Joanne prayed, "God, take him. He is nothing but a shell of the man he was." She realized, "I have nothing in common with Walt now. He has nothing on his mind except taking his drugs." Walt had become an addict. She stood by him and gave him loving care, but Walt's misery seemed endless. Still on Valentine's Day 2014, six months before he died, Walt told Joanne how grateful he was for the love she had given him for nearly 40 years.

In June, telling Joanne, "Before I die, I'm going to walk once again into the ocean by myself," he decided to have a second knee replacement. In July, following Walt's surgery, Joanne took him back to their home in Massachusetts to recuperate.

Coming to the End

The weekend of July 4, while Joanne ran an errand, Walt had a bad fall. He already had emphysema, his lung cancer had spread, and now he had a broken hip. His doctor said they should operate to make him more comfortable, told Joanne that Walt probably was not going to bounce back this time, and asked Walt whether he was prepared to die.

"Oh, goddamn, maybe I won't come out of it," Walt told Joanne. The look on his face said, "This is the final straw." The night before his last operation, Walt said, "Joanne, I loved you. I wasn't the best husband in the world but I tried."

When he opened his eyes in the recovery room, the disappointed look on his face said, "Oh, I'm still here." He was beyond being cared for at home now and had to go to a nursing home. Joanne set up a cot in his private room and slept by his bed for the next three weeks. There were times in the middle of the night, with his breathing labored and Walt so desperately in pain, when his opiates had to be given more often. This time, their priest friend administered the last rites. After spending 45 minutes talking with Walt, Father Ken told Joanne that her husband was at peace with facing death.

"A week before he died," Joanne recalls, "he put his arms up in the air and spoke to his brother, Bob, who had passed on some years before him." Walt called out, "Bob, I can see you. I can see you."

Walt was rushed from the nursing home to a hospital in a desperate breathing crisis. There, six days before he died, Walt told Joanne, "Close the crying room. Open the party room. Remember me with fun." Walt also said he wanted to go to their home now, in an ambulance. "The look on his face," Joanne explained, "said, 'Let's go end this.' It was a look that made it not feel so wrong for me to go choose a funeral home while he was still alive."

Joanne called Walt's three grown children and told them she was taking their dad home for hospice care. Recalling those last days, Joanne said, "Walt's children arrived three days before he died. He acknowledged their presence and mustered the energy to smile. They felt he knew they were there."

Two days before he died, Walt said something to Joanne that has haunted her since: "Joanne, we're going to have a long talk. But right now I'm going to the other side for a while." Joanne is still wondering, "What did he want to tell me? I've still got to figure out what he wanted me to know."

"He Was Finally Free"

On the day he died, Joanne sat close and watched his labored breathing. There was "a little puff of a breath at the last, and then Walt died," Joanne told me. "I was so relieved to look at his face, finally not tense and no longer gasping for every breath. He was finally free from having the air trapped in those diseased lungs. Finally free.

"When the staff member from the funeral home came, he treated Walt's body with such delicacy," Joanne continued, "as if Walt was his own father. Walt's face was left uncovered, and an American flag was draped across his chest. That's the memory I have of Walt being wheeled out of the house. He was at peace. Walt was a man who loved his country and he died in a peaceful state."

The day of the funeral, Joanne recalled, "I had total composure. Walt's portrait with his huge, wonderful smile and big blue eyes [was there for all to see], at the restaurant where everyone had lunch after the Mass. We passed the mike around among 80 people, and for a whole hour everyone wanted to tell stories. There was an open bar, the kids laughed and told stories. It was a huge and wonderful party. I could feel Walt just watching and celebrating. This is what his life was and who he really was."

Walt's children had been in the house with Joanne for 10 days by the time they left. "They each talked with their spouses. I didn't have anyone with whom to share what I was feeling." Without a husband for the first time in 40 years, "I was alone. I cried and cried. They were tears of grief but mostly what I felt was utter relief. It was a strange kind of crying—endless amounts of fluid were released in relief. For three or four days, I used towels, not tissues."

"Those last years were very hard for you," I said to Joanne. "How could you *not* feel enormous relief?"

"I have no regrets," Joanne replied. "I didn't hold back one moment of giving to Walt." She felt guilty saying it, Joanne told me, "but there were times when what I prayed to God was, 'End this now. There is not much more that You can give me that I can bear.'"

Joanne remembers that "there was a constant stream of people who came to visit." Family members and friends stayed a week or longer, including Joanne's nieces, nephews, Walt's children, and others who came back to celebrate Joanne's seventieth birthday. "When they left," she recalls, "I wondered, how much can I keep distracting myself?" Feelings of emptiness hit her hard.

One of her closest friends, Sharon, "a recovery room nurse with a huge heart, came at the perfect time to stay a week and help pack up and donate Walt's clothes." Sharon then accompanied Joanne on her first trip back to South Carolina after Walt's death in Massachusetts. This was the place in the sun—where Joanne and Walt shared countless good times. Just inside the condominium's threshold, Joanne burst into tears. Sharon held her and said, "Just cry, Joanne. Don't hold it in." In her friend's arms, Joanne cried and cried some more. Everything in sight and everything she touched triggered feelings of sadness. "Just having Sharon with me when I took Walt's ice tea pitcher out of the refrigerator helped so much."

Joanne recalled how, "from the time we were married, when his kids were young and living with their mother most of the time, Walt and I just talked and talked. We'd spend two hours in conversation over dinner. It was as if we'd had a 35-year-long date." Now, everything in that condo was a reminder of "loving Walt and losing him, piece by piece, in those last difficult years."

As she sought to move from the grief of losing the love of her life, and the relief that those awful years of Walt's suffering and her own distress were over, Joanne wondered, "What will be the meaning of the rest of my life?" How would life become purposeful and fulfilling again? After nine months, she said to herself, emphatically, "Well, I'm not going to spend the rest of my life looking at four walls!"

She thought of her own mother. "After losing two husbands, my mother found a companion and they did many things together, including going polka dancing . . . Maybe *I* can find a companion to talk with over dinner."

ANTICIPATORY MOURNING AND FEELINGS OF RELIEF

Family members, friends, and acquaintances often don't understand how a widow or widower can even think of dating sooner than a year or two after their spouse's death. People often judge and stigmatize what they don't understand. In this case, what is not understood is that *we often grieve for a long time* before *our loved one dies*, and thus our primary emotional reaction after the death is a profound sense of relief. Our loved one is no longer suffering and our caregiving work—often utterly exhausting—is now complete. In Joanne's case and for many others whose loved one dies a prolonged death from cancer, Alzheimer's disease, or another type of dementia or illness, often the mourning process is shortened by the fact that so much of one's grief work has already been done.

We also know from bereavement research that having shared a loving relationship makes you more likely to know that the person you've lost would *want* you to find happiness again in loving friendships or an intimate relationship. Think of the people *you* love, whether your spouse or children or siblings, and consider what *you* will want if you are the first to die. Won't you hope for your dearest loved ones to grieve for a time but then find ways to move beyond sadness to live fulfilling lives?

As a doctoral student and young therapist studying grieving people, I thought I knew a lot of things that now seem awfully presumptuous and have turned out to be dead wrong. Two of the "ah-ha!" realizations gleaned from the bereavement work I've done over the decades are that (1) mourning is a very individual thing, unique to each person in its healing stages, and (2) the older we are, the more quickly our period of sorrow needs to progress—while there is still time to cherish life and living.

Yes, the grief and healing process is shorter the older we get, at least our period of mourning *needs* to be shorter in our later adult lives. Because we have less remaining time to live, it helps no one, honors no one, serves no good purpose to grieve so long that you essentially die, too!

One of my colleagues was 56 when she felt a large lump in her breast as she sat with her 57-year-old husband in the hospital while he was being treated for cancer. Fearing she was going to lose him soon, Marla focused on caring for her husband, postponed seeing her own doctor, and didn't learn that she herself had a late-stage cancer until after Marvin died. Within a few months of becoming a widow, Marla started to date. She was a young-looking and attractive woman who had always dressed in stylish clothes, and some people at our workplace commented on how "good" she looked. They seemed to imply that Marla "wasn't showing a proper respect" for her husband. But Marla knew her own diagnosis—and, besides that, it was nobody's business but her own, if and when she decided to seek male companionship. The critics were hushed and hopefully felt ashamed for being so judgmental when Marla died only about a year after Marvin. I knew the couple well and how devoted they were to one another and to their adult children. Marla was not disrespecting their daughters or dishonoring her beloved husband; she was just "catching some meaningful living" while there was still time.

We never know what others' hearts are feeling or the challenges others are facing. None of us knows how much time *someone else* needs to mourn or when it's time to move forward. It is enough of a challenge to figure out for ourselves, when *we* lose a loved one, what is the "time for everything" described by the biblical writer of Ecclesiastes: "*For everything there is a season, and a time for every matter under heaven: a time to be born and a time to die . . . a time to weep, and a time to laugh; a time to mourn, and a time to dance . . .*"

SAM AND HIS WIFE

She was the woman he loved from the time he was 20 and remembers lovingly still. He will always love her. Lorraine was "a spark plug, with a lively personality, and I was enthralled with her," Sam told me. He is 73 now, a widower who looks back with fresh insight on their life together.

Their wedding followed a three-year courtship. Two girls and a boy arrived within 30 months of each other. A "caboose" daughter was to be born 17 years later, when Lorraine was forty-one.

They wanted to announce the news of this "miracle" pregnancy to the three siblings all at once. When the eldest came home from college for spring break, Sam and Lorraine said, "We have a surprise. Guess what it is?"

The college girl spoke first, "Oh, we're going skiing!"

The boy said, "We're having shrimp for dinner!"

And the younger daughter exclaimed, "I'm finally getting my horse!"

Lorraine, three months along, delicately lifted up her blouse and pulled out a tiny Christmas stocking for the fireplace mantel. It read, "BABY." Sam thinks it was his son who reacted first, "Oh, sh--!"

"A Wonderful Life"

"I had a wonderful life," Sam said warmly as we laughed together over the siblings' three guesses. "Back when Lorraine and I went for the church's premarital counseling," he continued, "the advice we got was, 'Keep it hot and never go to bed mad.' In 38 years of marriage, if we had an argument, we got over it before bedtime. There was never resentment carried over from yesterday or last Christmas, never a grudge carried from [decades earlier]. We argued, then—BINGO!—it was over with."

I asked Sam how they got on so well, after he'd said that Lorraine was such a spitfire. She verbally confronted her kids' teachers at PTA meetings and honked impatiently at other cars, described by Sam as "road rage before people called it that." On one such occasion, he told her, "I'm going to ride in my truck instead of your car. I don't want to get shot!"

Sam said he understood Lorraine and attributed her feisty personality to having been the third girl in her family before the long-awaited arrival of her parents' first and only son. Perhaps it was the middle child syndrome of having had a baby brother who garnered so much attention that made her "the kind of person who protected her turf, like a mother lion," Sam surmised. "If she felt she was right about something, she wouldn't back down."

Maybe she was just born with spirit and spunk. Regardless, Sam enjoyed and loved her just the way she was. "We were best friends," he went on. "There was nobody in my life who was a better friend. I worked long hours and had to be away a lot. She was a full-time stay-at-home mom. She never complained if I was late for dinner. She always had my back and was extremely loyal."

A Diagnosis of Cancer

Lorraine had always taken good care of herself, which was part of why her diagnosis was such a shock. "She played tennis, took two walks a day, maybe smoked a couple of cigarettes and had a couple of glasses of wine a week. She lived a healthy lifestyle."

Her doctor noticed that Lorraine's white blood count had been going down over several years. A medical test, drawing bone marrow from her hip, led to the alarming diagnosis. "Lorraine was at my office, on the phone in another room," Sam recalls. "She hung up and said, 'They've told me I have cancer.' We were to go to the doctor's office to hear the details in two or three days."

The couple was told the grim news by a young physician seemingly lacking empathy and basic communication skills. Sam recalls the scene with disgust. "He came in to talk to Lorraine and me, with a blank face, as if to sell us a new car battery. The doctor said, 'This is hard. You have an incurable disease. It's called multiple myeloma. Your life expectancy is 36 months.' Then he shook our hands and out the door he went!"

Lorraine was 54 "when we were diagnosed." It was clearly *their* cancer to deal with and not Lorraine's alone. It would belong to the whole family, yet it would have perhaps the most profound effect on 11-year-old Erin, the only child still at home and especially close to her mother. Too young to grasp the grim reality of her mother's prognosis, over the next seven years she was present at, and an unwilling participant in, her parents' jarring roller coaster ride of hopes uplifted, then dashed, over the course of her mother's cancer treatments.

On the brink of puberty, Erin was right at the stage of development when a daughter most needs her mother. While her parents fought to save Lorraine's life, Erin also needed their help to navigate the challenges of adolescence.

"Mom kept things pretty even," Erin told me, many years later. "Her strength became my strength." But her mother's bravery wasn't something a daughter so young could maintain, 30-year-old Erin now acknowledges: "I was in denial. I didn't have the tools to cope." A sensitive girl, Erin became depressed in middle school. Tormented by bullies, she had thoughts of suicide. Her mother was a good listener, kind and supportive, yet probably unaware of just how dreadfully unhappy Erin was feeling day after day at school.

"After we were diagnosed," Sam continued, "Lorraine and I still laughed, played golf, traveled, and spent time with friends." Even on their way home from hearing the bad news, they visited a close friend who was within days of dying from cancer. Oddly, among the five couples in their group of best friends, four of the husbands would lose their wives to cancer. Lorraine would be the fourth to die. "We continued to enjoy ourselves as a family and together as much as possible, traveled to weddings out of town, and visited friends on the West Coast," Sam remembers. "But I could look at Lorraine's face and see that she had a gun to the back of her head."

Second Opinions, Second Chances

They traveled to the MD Anderson Cancer Center in Texas, the Mayo Clinic in Minnesota, and the Cleveland Clinic in Ohio. Each one confirmed the diagnosis that they didn't want to hear. At one of Boston's renowned medical facilities, Lorraine underwent a 20-day hospitalization for a treatment that involved drawing out and radiating some of her bone marrow, then placing it back into her spine. For about 36 months, Lorraine's white blood cell count responded well to the radiation. "Her hair grew back," Sam remembers, "and our quality of life was pretty good. She never complained." With his practical approach, fitting for a certified public accountant, Sam's attitude was, "Let's hunker down and get through this as best as we can."

In October 2000, Lorraine was terribly sick again. She was also a candidate for a bone marrow transplant, and her sister was a perfect match. Told the cost was going to be a million dollars, Sam's heart sank. He had no idea where he was going to get that kind of money, "but I was going to keep her alive," he said. Because her cancer was at an early stage and the transplant could put her into long-term remission or even be a cure, Sam's health insurance policy covered the cost. "The disease was put into a pretty strong remission," Sam recalled. "However, our hopes were eventually dashed when Lorraine's body rejected the transplant. Her strength was sapped and depression set in. Every day she coped constantly with a dry mouth, dry eyes, and rashes on her face."

Sam had to tell himself and Lorraine, "We have a challenge here. Let's respond to the challenge," he went on. "My wife never cared for taking pills, but now she had to take 20 to 40 pills every day. As a person who likes math, I counted up that she took 75,000 to 100,000 pills in the seven years she lived with cancer," surviving more than twice as long as the first doctor had predicted.

Feeling the Grief

"Just a year before her mother was diagnosed, Erin had been so unbelievably accomplished that she was the wonder of the neighborhood," her dad told me. "Erin was the child about whom people said, 'How can she be good at everything?' But by the time she was a senior in high school," Sam went on, "Erin was defiantly breaking all the rules, and Lorraine had no discipline at all. There was conflict in the whole household."

By August 2003, "our oldest child was married and had four children," Sam explained, bookmarking this pivotal period in the family's life. "The next daughter was in the process of adopting a child from China, our boy was dating and planning to get married, and Erin was heading off to the University of Massachusetts Amherst."

That October, "Lorraine wanted to have an upbeat sixtieth birthday party. All the sibs came and we had a great time. Erin was home from college for the first time in her freshman year, and Lorraine wouldn't let Erin do anything, not even take a dish to the sink or carry the trash out. Erin knew her mother was going to die, and Lorraine felt tremendously guilty that she was dying and leaving her youngest child without a mom."

Erin came home for the summer. "Like many others—whose moms were *not* dying—I had started smoking a lot of pot in college," she told me, looking back. "I've always been rebellious, and I liked having the freedom to hang out with my friends."

Her dad knew she was partying and smoking marijuana, and he was "unhappy that Erin's grades weren't up to par." Under tremendous stress, Sam did the only thing he knew to do then: he came down hard on Erin. "I was going crazy," he told me. Once that summer, he took Erin to the hospital for an emergency appendectomy in the middle of the night. Hours after the surgery, she was "out running around with her friends." Sam was exhausted and short of sleep, and Erin was not acting the way he felt she should when she didn't spend more time with her dying mother. He was utterly perplexed and feeling furious about Erin's behavior: "She hadn't even told her friends that her mother was sick."

"I was repressing my feelings," Erin realizes now, 12 years later. "I didn't have the capacity to absorb what the truth was." Her always-nurturing, loving mother was dying. And the parent she was going to be left with was being "harsh and judgmental," in her eyes. Like most 18-year-olds facing an impending and unbearable loss, Erin was virtually without insight into her escapist behaviors. Smoking pot also was something she enjoyed. "I rarely ever did mourn. I just took on a tough outlook," she recalls.

Acknowledging that "my mother's death did throw me off course, and explains why I still have trouble coping with many situations and needed eight years to finish college," Erin understands now why she has battled depression. Unfortunately, when she sought medical help, Erin felt the prescriptions she tried throughout the years "caused more harm than good," and she quit taking them. An intelligent, resilient person, Erin says, "I maintain a healthy lifestyle by exercising, eating raw foods, drinking purified water, and by using alternative medicine and holistic therapies to keep me at an optimal sense of well-being." Since graduating from college, her passions include loving music, being concerned for the environment, and finding ways to be a voice for people who are disadvantaged or unable to speak for themselves.

RESOURCES FOR CHILDREN FACING LOSS

One of the encouraging trends in health care is attention paid to the emotional needs of patients and families dealing with life-threatening illness and death. There are child psychologists, clinical social workers, and certified art therapists able to help young children express their grief through play therapy, crafts, or art. Children facing the loss of one of their parents, with early professional help, may be spared a battle with depression that can go on for years. When needed, your community mental health center, nearby hospital, state psychological association, or child's physician can recommend an appropriate child therapist.

Coming To—and Controlling—the End

"Lorraine was on a water slide," Sam realized, "and it's hard when you're on a water slide to turn around and go back." During that summer, Lorraine decided to forgo one last attempt to extend her life with an experimental regimen of chemotherapy drugs her oncologist recommended. She didn't want to undergo another hospitalization and treatment ordeal that would buy her only a little more time. "She'd always liked her hair, was glad it had grown back, and she didn't want to lose it again," Sam recalls. "The doctors radiated her spine, so she was not in a great deal of pain. The only medications she had were antidepressants."

There was so little that Lorraine could still control in her life. Keeping her hair was one of those things, and how she would spend her last few weeks was another. "Once her doctor warned that death would likely happen within three weeks," Sam recalls with admiration, "Lorraine decided she wanted to let the kids and her friends know that her time left was very short. Seventy-five people came to the house and sat by her hospital bed. Friends would come with lunches and she would eat with them. She had lost so much weight, she was all shriveled up like dried fruit, but her mind was sharp. She had guests every day and enjoyed every minute of it. The children kept taking turns coming back to the house. They sat on the bed with her and laughed and talked together."

It was only half an hour's drive to his office, Sam went on. "There was a supportive crew there, though, and I worked fewer and fewer hours. But work was good for me and Lorraine knew it. She said, 'I'm fine. If I need you, I'll call.' I did the cooking at home, and she was slow but up and around until two weeks before she died. Until then, we walked and talked although she was losing her strength."

Lorraine's hospital bed was downstairs so Sam made a bed with blankets and slept on the floor beside her. "I didn't want her to suffer," he said, "and I was up at one point for 36 hours straight, when she had periods of gasping for breath. Finally I got so tired that I couldn't move and went upstairs to sleep, just to catch a little rest. The toughest thing was when I came downstairs. I felt so bad because she'd gotten herself tangled in her bedding and catheter. I told her I was sorry that I hadn't heard her ring the bell but she didn't say anything. She understood. I probably should have had a portable bed to sleep on. And we probably should have had someone there to help us full time, but she didn't want that."

During the last 10 or 12 days, hospice nurses came, and "they were wonderful," Sam remembers. "Then in that final 72-hour phase, when Lorraine didn't want food or water, I braced myself and just sat there listening to her labored breathing. I felt so depressed. It was a terrible time." When Lorraine's breathing had changed and suddenly stopped, Sam had said to himself, "Please don't come back." He knew that she was ready to die. "She was so weak that she couldn't lift a finger," he said. "I was relieved that her suffering was over."

The "Survival Mode"

Erin was 18 and in the second week of her sophomore year when the urgent call came. Arriving home, she said, "Hi, Mom," to her mother lying on a hospital bed in the living room and kept right on going to the safety of her bedroom. When the terrible loss she had been dreading from the age of 11 was near, she was frightened and devastated, having tried so hard to will away this horrible day. Erin's unconscious response was driven by a combination of denial and distraction. She loved her mother, was overwhelmed with grief, and was coping in the best and only ways she knew how.

Sometimes we human beings just go into "survival mode"—simply blocking out an approaching loss and not allowing ourselves to acknowledge it. Erin had many strengths, even when very young. For her, and many other children, blocking out a looming loss is often the defense mechanism that best makes it possible to stand strong, at least until old enough to handle intense grief. We get by using whatever ways of coping we can manage at the time.

Like Erin, her siblings, and their mother, Sam was trying to get by as best he could. The head of the family, holding things together to be strong for Lorraine, he was under enormous stress, month after month for those seven years. He hadn't shared his worry and grief along the way, "not wanting to burden the children," although he was able to talk with some of his friends. "After Lorraine died," he told me, "I had a terrible time with depression and my body folded under the stress."

Only 10 days after her death, Sam was heading to work when he suffered intense pain with his sciatic nerve. "It was so severe that I pulled into a parking lot and couldn't drive. Finally I drove back home and literally crawled up the stairs of our colonial house and flopped into bed. Lorraine's oncologist happened to call right then to see how I was doing. She said she'd get an appointment for me right away with someone who could give me an epidural for pain. The stress was eating me up."

After having had a normal PSA that June before Lorraine died in September, Sam explained, "in December my numbers had doubled and I was diagnosed with an aggressive form of prostate cancer. I had surgery in April, plus four subsequent surgeries, and a stroke over that next decade."

Surviving Stress and Moving On

When friends who are losing their wives call him for advice and ask him what to expect, Sam tells them, "You must know yourself and appreciate that stress eats at you like the cancer that eats at your spouse. Expect that you might get sick yourself, so *watch your own health*."

Sam also tells other men, "When it comes to your wife's illness, it also helps to know what to expect. The human brain can take care of anything as long as there are no surprises, and if you have time to absorb it. I tell doctors to give me all the bad news on the front end, *then* look at the positive options."

Support groups help too, Sam says, having learned in his journey through personal crisis that "bonds develop in bad times, not good." Mourning involves digging down deep, and the support group that he joined helped him look back over a lot of sorrowful memories, ponder what could have been different, and realize that he probably couldn't have changed anything. "Stress is brutal and so is mourning," Sam continued, but over time he came to the place where "I feel blessed that Lorraine lived as long as she did."

He is also blessed with a lot of friends, bonds developed in good times *and* bad, men with whom he often went out to lunch. "I'm convinced that Lorraine told them all to look out after me after she was gone. Our friends would call and they called for several years after her death."

Later on, "I had my wife's friends wanting me to be happy and trying to fix me up to date someone acceptable to them. I called them the 'posse,' and I made some mistakes with all these fix-ups, sometimes going out with a woman for too long when the chemistry wasn't there. I wasn't going to 'settle,' and I did irritate some people I didn't keep dating. Plus I had my own health issues."

JOANNE AND SAM: GOING FORWARD

A theme throughout this chapter is that it is important to move on with one's own life. Sometimes that happens in ways that seem like a Hollywood script, as in the case of Joanne and Sam, who found each other after the deaths of Walt and Lorraine.

In 2015, Sam met someone special through a dating site. This woman met his three criteria: "She had to be a Catholic. She had to be conservative. And she had to know what a bogey was." That woman was Joanne. She fit the first two categories and, being a golfer, she definitely knew that a bogey is one over par. The added bonus was that Joanne is an attractive, interesting, and bright woman. Their story speaks to second chances for caregivers who have survived loss—and the courage it takes to embrace those chances.

At the age of 70, Joanne joined a dating website. "There were faces popping up right away," she recalled. "I answered a list of questions, and, three days later, there was a man named Sam who wrote to me. He said, 'It looks like we have a lot in common. Let's have lunch.'"

Joanne wondered, "Am I ready to do this? Well, I like to play golf and maybe there's someone I could talk with about losing my husband," she decided. "I just have to move on."

Joanne and Sam exchanged several one- or two-liner e-mails. They planned to meet for lunch, but Sam got cold feet and canceled. "When we finally did meet, I learned that Sam had a business in Massachusetts just 10 blocks from our house, a place that Walt and I had passed by often," Joanne remembers. "Walt used to say, as we drove by, 'Someday we should stop in there.'"

"Sam is a warm, gentle, understanding soul." Especially meaningful has been the fact that "we have cried together and share our grief over losing our spouses."

"But Walt wasn't even dead a year and I was feeling nervous," Joanne went on. "Walt's kids thought it was way too soon for me to be dating. There is a social stigma to moving on not long after your loved one's death," she realized. "But I have asked myself, whose calendar are we on now?"

Joanne, like the rest of us, didn't know what was in store for her, but she moved ahead into life, as did Sam, and eventually their lives came together.

Almost from the beginning, Joanne noticed the easy way that she and Sam were able to talk together about the spouses each had loved and lost, and so much more. Joanne's father had died of multiple myeloma, just as Sam's wife had. Joanne had survived breast cancer and melanoma in her 40s and 50s. Sam had survived prostate cancer, heart problems, and a mild stroke in his 60s. Sam described the process of their getting to know each other as "everybody comes with baggage—here's mine. When you're 22 or 25," he said, "you come with a clean slate. At 73 and 71, there's a plethora of issues: health, family, friends, and different interests." Still, Sam "knew quickly, within weeks, that she was the one I'd been waiting for." Five months after their first date, he proposed.

Although Joanne's response was, "We can't talk about a future until you've met my family," she had begun to fall in love the third time they met in person. "It was on a date that lasted nine hours," she recalls sweetly. "Sam kissed me for the first time then, and I realized that I want to be kissed by this man for the rest of my life."

But, in late adulthood, love relationships are "much more complicated," Sam acknowledges. As he sees it, "A couple has to combine two lives that are already 100 percent full, and each gets to keep only 50 percent of all the people among their friends and family."

Whether Joanne sees marriage as requiring letting go of so many relationships valued over a lifetime remains to be seen. There are many things they need to talk about before more big decisions are made, Joanne realizes, because "we will have a different marriage than either of us had before."

Of course there will be challenges ahead, but "there is nothing better than a good marriage," Joanne continued. Sharing the joys of being in love again and building a rewarding life together is exactly what Joanne and Sam have wholeheartedly begun to do.

Life Is Too Short Not to Live It Fully

Joanne thinks back to when she was 55 and had a profound spiritual experience following her surgery, radiation, and chemotherapy treatments for breast cancer. Realizing that she had been given another chance to live, Joanne took a deep breath and prayed, "Okay, God, you're giving me my life back. What do you want me to do?" Years later, "Seeing Walt die gave me another vivid reminder that we are all mortal."

Sam cherishes "Joanne's genuineness, sincerity, lack of pretension, and comfortableness with herself." He counts himself lucky because "she is a lovely person in every way. She has nice friends and a wonderful family, a strong core and support system."

"We're both blessed with wonderful families and friends," Sam goes on. "At the same time, we are a new family and it's very easy to be put on a guilt trip to have the same holiday gatherings and same vacation times."

Joanne most values how "Sam lights up a room and just brings joy to everybody. He loves people, is outgoing, very giving, and has a genuine concern and devotion to family. He is a good man who will go out of his way to be a kind person."

At 71 and 73, Joanne and Sam have challenges ahead as they endeavor to blend their extended families, combine their homes, and maintain ties with lifelong friends; and none of these changes is likely to be easily navigated.

Nonetheless, Joanne and Sam each delight in the good fortune of having found each other. They both expect to live happily together, until death parts them.

Embracing the Future

Change is an inevitable reality of human life. Joanne and Sam, Joyce, and my friend Marla all know in their hearts that this is true and offer us wisdom hard won through grief. We have to be able to go forward with our lives after we lose people we love. To live well means finding a renewed sense of meaning in life and opportunities for new adventures—for as long as our health and life circumstances allow it. Challenges come with change, yet by taking chances, including taking the chances that always come with falling in love, developing new friendships, or finding other ways to live purposefully, our lives will continue to be interesting.

In his book *Chancing It*, Ralph Keyes writes that Americans associate taking a risk with doing something dramatic. What may be a far more courageous act for many people, he states, would be to quietly attune ourselves to our own needs and fears, and bring to the surface "fears of commitment, responsibility, and rootedness." Staying put, for example, committing oneself to a marriage partner, career, or family, or making some commitment to something that is important to us may be far riskier than a more sensational action. In the final analysis, Keyes says, it is the "spirit of being adventuresome" that provides excitement, and it is the ability to make and keep deep commitments that brings happiness.[2]

What Kind of an "Old Person" Will I / Will You Become?

It is time for us to let go of both our fantasies about eternal youth and our fears of getting older, and to find the beauty of what it means to age well.
 —Joan Chittister, *The Gift of Years*

Thinking ahead to growing older, I don't know anyone who doesn't fervently hope not to develop Alzheimer's, dementia from another cause, or a severe physical disability. Most of us would wish to live to 90, 95, or 100—*if* we could remain reasonably healthy, especially mentally. We want to continue to make our own decisions, without relying on others to care for our most basic needs and then one day, with a minimum of suffering, simply die very old, and very peacefully, surrounded by our loved ones.

FACING OUR WORST FEARS

Frankly, while interviewing caregivers and researching this book, I struggled with my own age-related anxiety and fear. Both my mother and maternal grandmother had Alzheimer's with increasingly severe memory problems and other impairments, from 85 to 89, the age at which they each died. Having been a heavy cigarette smoker when young, and knowing that smokers have twice the risk of dementia, I hope that I quit in time and have enough offsetting healthy lifestyle behaviors to save my arteries and brain!

Genetic risks for Alzheimer's disease play a role in our vulnerability to developing the dreaded dementia, as do other risk factors that include diabetes, high blood pressure and heart disease, obesity, a history of head injuries or strokes, untreated severe depression, unmitigated long-term stress, or exposure to environmental toxins. Early-onset Alzheimer's and Huntington's disease (far less common types of dementia), and a few others *are* caused by one's genetic inheritance. *Still, researchers and gerontologists agree that what shapes our destiny in old age—in most cases, more than our genes—starts with a healthy blood pressure and diet, regular exercise plus a strong social support system, and includes some combination of lifelong learning, positive beliefs and attitudes toward aging, a sense of meaning and purpose in our lives, and good habits for coping with stress.*

There are no guarantees for any of us, of course. We can only choose to live with optimism, fend off ageist stereotypes, take care of ourselves as best we can, and make lifestyle changes and preparations that maximize our chances of aging well as long as possible. Most of us won't make *all* of the lifestyle changes listed above but we can make *many* of them—especially getting any needed medical treatment for high blood pressure and cholesterol, walking 30 minutes a day, and staying active mentally. *We can build and plan for the best life within reach.*

In this chapter I'll be talking about what we can learn from the literature on aging and from the examples of people who are "aging successfully." Hopefully, we can significantly increase *our* chances of living well as close to our deaths as possible. Earlier in this book I told the story of a woman I interviewed who is still living a meaningful life at the age of 108; here I will be sharing the mostly brief but powerful stories of people from 64 to 94 whose lives demonstrate vitality and purpose.

As noted in earlier chapters, your mind-set—attitude, or whatever you call it—can make a tremendous difference, to you, the ones you care for, and the ones who will care for you. For most of us, this means giving up destructive myths about aging, called ageism. We stand to pay a high price for buying into ageism, but we don't have to. We can live happier, fuller lives if we don't.

"STEREOTYPE THREAT"

Simply put, "stereotype threat," a concept that has been widely studied, means that we can very easily become the victim of aging stereotypes that we aren't even aware of, "messages" that we pick up unconsciously *and* adopt. These implicit ageist messages, along with the countless and more obvious negative stereotypes from the media and the responses of people who don't know us but respond to us with age prejudice, have an alarmingly effective impact. The research findings are clear: if we buy into those stereotypes, we literally will not hear as well, remember as well, think as clearly, or stand as straight, walk as fast, or feel as self-worthy as we will if we recognize, resist, and reject those ageist stereotypes. We truly and actually can bring about the self-fulfilling prophecy of feeling, acting, and appearing to others "old" before our time![1]

"Most older people . . . say they feel younger than they look and than they actually are," writes Laura E. Berk, in *Development Through the Lifespan.* "In several investigations," she reports, "75-year-olds reported feeling about 15 years younger!"[2] Furthermore, in "happiness surveys around the world," explains physician Henry Lodge, a professor at Columbia University Medical School, a majority of people 70 and older said they are as happy as they have ever been. "When Americans over 65 were asked, 'What were the best years of your life?' more than 50 percent said, 'Right now!'"[3]

You would never know—if you watch much television—that more and more of us are not just living longer; we are living healthier, more active, more satisfied, and more fulfilling lives. It can be very difficult to think of late adulthood (65–79) or old age (80–100+) as something *good*, given the frequency of media portrayals and TV advertisements for chair lifts, catheters, hearing aids, medications for blood clots and dementia, and the MedicAlert devices supposedly needed for those poor women writhing around on the floor calling for help when no one is answering!

Here are the facts: glasses, hearing aids, and medicine are not "age-related" means of assistance. Many young people depend on them as well. It is unfortunate that they've become part of the ageist mythology. Furthermore, older people who use them usually function just as well as those who don't. Unfortunately, many medical and other companies' advertisements intentionally use stereotypes of "all alone and anxious, fearful and frail" elders to sell their products. Depression and feelings of loneliness are significantly *less* common when we are older than when we were younger. Most forms of dementia are *un*common before age 85 and only affect fewer than half of those who are 85 and older. By taking control of our attitudes and behavior and not passively assuming that deterioration and disability are inevitabilities, we can stay younger longer. We can eat healthier and exercise, stay in close contact with our friends and family, adapt our living environment to remain as active as possible, and adopt a lifelong love of learning.

In their research publication, "Hearing Decline Predicted by Elders' Stereotypes," Becca Levy and her colleagues at Yale University found that "age stereotypes influence older individuals' sensory perception," which results in "a significantly heightened cardiovascular response to stress," elevating certain stress chemicals (called cytokines), which "could negatively affect hearing."[4]

My own experience drives home this lesson. My father and brother both had hearing problems by age 60 or earlier. For them, it made sense because of the thousands of hours each spent riding a very loud John Deere tractor while planting wheat and pulling plows, mowers, and bailing machines. In those days, America's farmers didn't have headphones with music to enjoy while working the fields or tractors with comfortable air-conditioned cabins. Daddy and Vaughn were also hunters. It's no wonder they lost so much hearing from the blasts and reverberations of their shotguns and from the "poppin' Johnny" noise of our 1950s tractor. Although I didn't have their noise pollution exposure, I somehow got the idea, around the age of 65, that I was having an age-related hearing loss. I was straining to hear my college students' questions from the back rows of my classrooms. When, after several years of attributing the "hearing problem" to "getting older," I went to a medical specialist for testing and was surprised to learn that my hearing is "just fine"! Only then did I allow myself to accept the explanation that the noisy heating and air-conditioning units in the back of the rooms *are* noisy—so, of course, the students speaking from back there are harder to hear. *I had bought into the stereotyped notion that aging inevitably brings with it impaired hearing!* Now, unapologetically, I just ask those on the back row to speak up.

Still, hearing impairments *are* more common in late adult life, affecting approximately 12 percent of women and 17 percent of men by age 75 and nearly 60 percent of men and nearly 50 percent of women by age 85.[5] Getting your hearing tested and using hearing aids when needed has been shown in recent studies to significantly improve cognitive function,[6] slow down the progression of dementia symptoms, and reduce the kinds of paranoid ideas that commonly are experienced by elders who misinterpret what others are saying or think people are whispering.

Buying into ageist stereotypes without questioning their validity can make a profound difference in how we live our lives: "Self-stereotypes of aging" are the age stereotypes we internalize "several decades before becoming old," explains Becca Levy of the Yale School of Public Health. Remarkably, a recent study led by Levy has shown that "individuals who hold negative beliefs about aging are more likely to have brain changes associated with Alzheimer's disease." Examining data from America's most comprehensive and lengthy scientific study of aging, Levy and her colleagues saw in the brain scans of people with negative beliefs about aging "a greater decline in the volume of the hippocampus, a part of the brain crucial to memory. Reduced hippocampus volume is an indicator of Alzheimer's disease." The researchers also studied brain autopsies showing that study participants who held negative beliefs about aging in midlife, documented about 28 years before they died, at death had "a significantly greater number of the plaques and tangles" known to be indicators of Alzheimer's disease! Says Levy, "We believe it is the stress generated by the negative beliefs about aging that individuals sometimes internalize from society that can result in pathological brain changes." Researchers like these at Yale hope this research demonstrates "that these negative beliefs about aging can be mitigated and positive beliefs about aging can be reinforced, so that the adverse impact is not inevitable."[7]

Contrary to the stereotype that "older people live in the past," writes psychologist Laura Berk, "research consistently reveals no age differences exist in total quantity of reminiscing!" Also, while a survey of older adults showed that "30 to 40 percent had been ignored, talked down to, or assumed to be unable to hear or understand well because of their age," Berk reports that "most older adults do not have a hearing loss great enough to disrupt their daily lives until after age 85 . . . [and that] even among people age 85 and older, only 30 percent experience visual impairment severe enough to interfere with daily living." In her textbook, used widely in college courses and published in 19 countries around the world, Berk goes on to cite an earlier longitudinal study by Levy and colleagues showing that older people who *refused to accept* negative age-related stereotypes "lived, on average, 7½ years longer than those with negative self-perceptions."[8]

Dr. Kurtinitis

"When I travel, the bus driver thinks he has to help me down the steps," says this college president. "Never in *my* mind am I an elderly person!" The driver means well but he sees a stereotype. *She* sees herself as a person who can't imagine retiring. "I'm having too much fun! If you derive joy from your job, why would you leave it?"

No one who actually knows Dr. Sandra Kurtinitis thinks of her as old, even though as of September 2017 her career in higher education spans half a century. At 72, she is the highly effective, widely esteemed president of the Community College of Baltimore County, with six campus locations serving more than 65,000 students. Four times recently, she was invited to the White House in recognition of the trend-setting institution she leads in Maryland. The college has won national awards for innovation and its evidence-proven success in opening doors for students socioeconomically disadvantaged and advantaged, for students needing additional academic support in order to succeed, and for students academically gifted.

Dr. Kurtinitis is a powerhouse of energy, wisdom, and leadership experience. She is a woman with things to do and places to go, blessed with the "people skills" to motivate and affirm excellence on the part of faculty, staff, and a richly diverse student population.

"A buoyant approach to life helps a person to stay young," she says, and goes on to mention Maggie Smith and Judi Dench (both 81), Jane Fonda (78), Dolly Parton (70), Meryl Streep (67), Alfre Woodard (63), and Hillary Clinton (68)—all still talented, working, and *not* talking as if their best years are over. "Dr. K." remembers glancing through the June/July 2016 issue of *AARP—the Magazine*, in which four-time Emmy winner Woodard is quoted: "Age is what you decide you want it to be. I am still in motion here."[9]

"I was getting to the point," Dr. Kurtinitis continued, "where I hated going down to the basement to use the exercise equipment, when my son said, 'Just do something physical three times a week, and you'll be fine.' So I walk a mile or two, follow a routine from a little Royal Canadian exercise book I've had for years, lift some weights, and work out on some level three days weekly. I lost 20 pounds two years ago, and doing all that keeps my body mobile and my mind clear."

When she sees a photo of herself, "I look old, yet I think of myself as not young but not old. My kids say I'm 70 going on 50, and that's how I feel."

Dr. Kurtinitis' perspective is that "I'm just a professional person who comes to work with joy and enthusiasm. My work life is at the absolute best point ever. Personally gratifying. All these years, I've been leading up to this point, and it's a wonderful apex. In a few years, I'll probably retire, but I'm not going to buy into those age-related stereotypes. Many people, at this stage in life, all they talk about is going to their doctor! If I feel my back is sore, I tell myself that I have a strong body. I'm not going to look at every little brown spot or ache and say, 'Uh oh, this means I'm old.' My doctor described me as 'a 70-year-old woman in the body of a 50-year-old,' and I heard that with real joy."

Wrapping up our conversation, Dr. K. returns to thoughts of her closest loved ones. "I draw great strength and joy from my family, but they are all happily engaged in their own service professions and scattered around the country.

My son is soon to be deployed to Afghanistan. There are no grandchildren yet. They were all here for the recent holiday. I don't need to see my three children every day to be happy. They are always with me, embedded in me."

AGING SUCCESSFULLY

For more examples of those who refuse to be bound by ageism and negative stereotypes, I look around at the people I know and admire. Their lives give a personal voice to the research I cite throughout this book. It's through my friends and my extended family—students I've taught, clients I've counseled, and the many people I've met in my everyday life—that I've learned what living well as older adults can be. Some have had to deal with tragedy during their lives and have overcome it, while others have been more fortunate. But they all are aging successfully. Let me introduce a few of them to you.

A Recent Widow, My Dad, and Dr. Carl Rogers

At 83, my brother's widow has moved to a senior living facility, but she still plays tennis three times a week with her girlfriends, all of them younger than she is. (Loving tennis as I do, I hope *I* can keep playing another ten or fifteen years!) My dad went hunting and won skeet shooting trophies until his eyesight slowly failed in his late 70s, but he continued to mow the lawn, manage finances, and walk two miles a day up to the age of 88. Even bedridden at 95, he enjoyed listening to music all day long until he died at 96. Early in my career, one of my most admired mentors, Dr. Carl Rogers, taught me when he was in his 70s and was still lecturing internationally, writing, and inspiring young psychologists at the age of 85. He was 87 when he died.

Burt and Linda

Having run two 26-mile marathons since turning 60, my friend Burt is an inspiration. At 68, he is up before dawn every Friday morning to run five miles to exercise and be a friend to men in a substance recovery and job program called Back on My Feet. Burt is a leader at his church, works full time as a civil engineer, is a loving husband and an actively involved grandfather, and enjoys cooking on the grill, reading nonfiction books, playing bridge, and following the Baltimore Orioles throughout the baseball season. He is a vibrant man, doing what he loves doing. Burt's wife, Linda, is a retired Food and Drug Administration scientist who lovingly babysits her grandchildren, teaches Sunday school, and enjoys gardening and playing bridge. She volunteers weekly as a tutor and reader to little kids who live in poor neighborhoods with few community resources, in underfunded schools in Baltimore City.

Ron

Ron and I have been friends since our late 20s / early 30s. We made many trips in a VW bus full of friends, driving to the Outer Banks of North Carolina. We were more or less "hippies" then, but both working in full-time jobs. Ron will be 70 years old by the time this book comes out, and he's a person I admire. In the navy, he was a mechanic working on diesel and jet engines in the Vietnam era, then a Toyota mechanic, then a Toro (lawnmower) specialist who taught other mechanics. Ron has had his obstacles and losses in life, but he has overcome them. In his last job, which he held for more than 30 years, he was the head groundskeeper at a private school for boys where he managed a million-dollar budget and a staff of crew members, repaired or replaced all the machines, and led the crew in every aspect of maintaining the 67-acre property. He retired from the top job two years ago, but he was asked to stay on part time and still works a 10 hour day, two days a week.

His philosophy is to "keep my *mind active*, my *body fit*, and to remain *morally adjusted*" (which, to Ron, means being honest with others and himself, and not blaming other people but accepting responsibility for his own actions). In semiretirement, he lifts weights and swims at an athletic club three days a week and enjoys vegetable gardening. He does more housework and cooking than he used to do, to make his wife's load lighter since she works full time. Once a week, Ron plays his guitar in a trio, playing a lot of Crosby, Stills, Nash, and Young; the Beatles; and Rolling Stones' favorites. He is a loyal and wonderful friend and loved by many. Ron and his wife, happy together in their second marriages, each are helping to finance her grandson through college. Ron likes working part time. "I'll never slow down," he says, "I want to stay active as long as I possibly can."

Jan

At 74, my friend Jan is a recently retired college professor who volunteers for Asylee Women Enterprises, an organization that offers housing, workshops, courses, and compassionate companionship to women who fled life-endangering abuse and violence to seek asylum in the United States. "I'm there two days a week," Jan explains, "organizing and teaching English as a Second Language." One day weekly, during the school year, Jan babysits and transports her five grandsons while her son and daughter-in-law are at work. Through her church, Jan helps raise funds for, and occasionally visits, a Haitian mountain village. As a certified master gardener, she volunteers 40 hours a year at farmers' markets and demonstration gardens. She keeps herself fit with exercise and taking yoga classes. Fluent in several languages, Jan and her husband occasionally travel to Europe, and they often entertain friends who live locally or visit from other countries.

Corporal Boccelli

Some people you just don't forget. I remember admiring him before I'd even met him after his Colonel told me that this policeman named Officer Boccelli—who had signed up for one of my psychology courses at the Baltimore County Police Training Academy—was a retired major in the army. He had started over at the lowest rung of the ladder, a rookie cop, after 20 years in military service that culminated in a base commander position, which was equivalent to being the mayor of a sizeable city.

That was 17 years ago. He is 60 now, soon to "retire" for a second time—again, after 20 years of service—and he is looking for a new job because "I don't envision retiring, and I enjoy being active." He'd like to become the director of security for an organization where he finally won't have to do shift work, can see more of his 30-year-old son, and can share more custody time with his five-year-old daughter.

Corporal Boccelli is a study in living thoughtfully, observing others' lives, and shaping his own path quite intentionally. "My father was in the military for 26 years, and a very kind, gentle man, not argumentative," he says. "Not one to take advantage of others, even if the opportunity presented itself. He aged well, but he took my mother's death very hard. In my work in law enforcement, I saw two extremes. One person's loved one would die, a huge dumpster would be in the driveway, and everything would be hauled away as if the dead person never existed. Another person's loved one died, and you'd go to the house 10 years later and see the deceased person's handbags still hanging up, and their underwear still in the drawer. That second way of handling grief—denial—is how my father was. It was sad to watch him go through such anguish."

Watching his father seem to lose his will to live made Corporal Boccelli decide "that life is not over at that point. It's incumbent on all of us to go on with living and stay actively involved in our activities, which are key factors for aging well."

When he went into law enforcement, Boccelli continued, "I had to eat a lot of humble pie. I went home at the end of that first week at the Police Training Academy, and my wife asked me what I learned. 'I learned to salute,' I told her. The second week, when she asked the same question, I said, 'I learned to march.' But what I really learned is that you do what you have to do to achieve your goal; you can't let your ego get in the way, you can't say 'that's beneath me,' you just have to take the high road."

Corporal Boccelli has thought a lot about how he wants to be remembered: "I just want to be thought of as a good person," he says. "Hopefully, if there's a day of reckoning, it will be said that I showed the same respect to a private, or a custodian, as to a general, that I never spoke down to someone because of rank or status." To this former military leader, now in law enforcement as his second career, a man with two master's degrees, what has always been gratifying is "working with the troops, whether soldiers or police officers." He supervises a squad of officers who handle 911 calls and "thoroughly enjoys the young people." From my own occasional interactions with Corporal Boccelli over the years, I have no doubt that the lesson to be learned from Boccelli's own life is getting through: "Treating everyone with respect and honor should be the cornerstone of everyone's character."

At the same time, he is very human. "Everybody has their day when they want to grab a milk box and strangle it," he says, with more than a little humor in his voice. "You have those days that are just so frustrating, but you work it out through exercise and get things back in perspective. Some things you have to accept: You can't change it, so why get upset over it, why spend time and energy getting frustrated over something you can't do anything about? 'It is what it is,' I try to say to myself."

Corporal Boccelli's goal is pretty basic: "I try to consciously appreciate every day—the sky, the trees, birds, and clouds—and be grateful that I can walk without assistance. I want my tombstone to say that I was thankful for what I have, not regretful for what I don't have."

Summing up another powerful perspective by which he tries to live, Corporal Bocelli says, "Each of us experiences adversity in our life. What's important is to take that adversity and learn something from it. If you learn from hard times and get a positive perspective, I believe it's conducive not only to your health but your sense of well-being, too. Some people, everything they say is negative. If you're a positive person, people want to be around you. Wine gets better with age, and I just want to become the best person I can be."

MAKING CHOICES

In some ways we do, and in other ways we don't, get to decide what *our* young old (ages 65–79) and old old (80–100+) years will look like. Staying active mentally and physically in our 50s, 60s, and 70s, however, greatly betters our chances for having minds that still function well and bodies that remain mobile in our 80s and 90s. People we consider role models in various ways can help us chart that intended course. Again, there are no guarantees for any of us, because a debilitating accident, illness, or fateful death can come in any number of ways, but what other choice makes sense, except to give life and living all the energy and optimism we can muster? We can *choose* to go full throttle, which is how our role models have been able to thrive.

What does it mean to live life well and grow older as a resilient person worthy of being looked to as a role model? In *my* mind, one would need to be a loving family person and loyal friend, a lifelong learner, a person of integrity who also remains physically active as long as possible, and someone who dies leaving behind lives aided or enriched by his or her compassion and concern.

Dorris

For nearly five decades, all the way to her recent death at the age of 91, a woman who taught me a great deal about successful aging was Dorris Moger Hoyle. She and her husband, Hal, were old enough to be my parents, but they always treated me as a peer and friend, even when I was a 22-year-old graduate student, working for the summer as a youth director in their church. The couple raised four good citizen children—two teachers, a dentist, and a nuclear power plant operator—each of them, like their parents, deeply involved in community leadership and service activities. When their son, Mark, died of cancer in his 40s, the family established a college scholarship in his name that was awarded for more than 20 years.

Dorris was a lifelong learner. In 1940, her mother made her quit college after seeing the pages devoted to human sexuality in Dorris' biology textbook! Instead, her parents paid for her to take the train daily from Valhalla into New York City to attend a secretarial school. At a dance for soldiers and sailors on leave during World War II, Dorris met the man from North Carolina who would be her husband for 55 years, then stationed with the US Navy in New York Harbor.

In the days of encyclopedias instead of the Internet, Dorris was always pulling a volume off the shelf to study up on a topic or enrich a conversation with interesting factual details. Her mind was wide open to seeking accurate information versus succumbing to bias or speculation. In the Jim Crow South of the 1940s, '50s, and '60s, where many local residents had huge paintings of the Confederate army's General Lee hanging in their living rooms, Dorris was an early advocate for racial equality. Ahead of her time, she also spoke up for women, gay people, and exploited mill workers. Dorris volunteered for more than 20 years as a guardian ad litem, advocating in court for one after another neglected or abused child. She volunteered for the Red Cross Bloodmobile and Meals on Wheels delivery, was a Girl Scout leader, and vice chair of the Lincoln County Democratic Party. With her husband, she enjoyed travel, Chinese furniture and art, boating, and entertaining at home. With her many friends, she played bridge, attended church events, and belonged to a book club. Dorris was an awesome cook and avid gardener, who canned vegetables for the family to enjoy year-round. She was a full-time mother at home for her children and a loving, generous "Gammy" to seven grandchildren and ten great-grandkids.

When I visited Dorris, we had wonderful conversations, staying up late to talk and have a glass or two of wine. Her genuine interest in my family and friends was palpable, and her encouragement as I pursued my education and career had a tremendously positive impact. My family was far away in Oklahoma, Texas, and California. It meant so much that Dorris came to hear me speak at events in North Carolina and sat on the floor feeding Cheerios to my firstborn as a toddler so I could nap. Later she babysat my girls while we traveled together on a book tour. Dorris came to Baltimore and to favorite southern beaches to share vacations with us. While I never felt much support from my family for my life's work, Dorris had a special shelf in her house for my books, which she gave away often and I replaced with regularity. A Yankee who learned to master southern hospitality, she always made my favorite dishes ahead of my visits, filling the refrigerator and cookie tins. Dorris loved me as part of her family—and what an intelligent, interesting, giving, and wonderful friend she was.

After her husband's death, Dorris continued to garden, visit friends, host bridal and baby showers for the grandchildren, and travel. She frequently exchanged e-mails with loved ones and still hosted the large family's holiday dinners. As her health failed and eyesight worsened, Dorris was able to continue to live alone in her own home, thanks to frequent visits from her helpful children and their spouses, who loved her, too.

Despite having *many* medical problems in the last 10 years of her life, Dorris remained active. She dressed herself attractively, did her own cooking, and washed her own clothes. Once her husband of 50 years had passed away, the ever-innovative Dorris made the clean bed sheets last two weeks instead of one by sleeping on the left side of the bed the first week and on the right side of the bed the next!

Being tethered to an oxygen tank didn't slow her down much at all. She just stretched out a 100-foot-long cord carrying oxygen from her bedroom, through the living room, dining area, kitchen, and onto her front porch or into the garage. She carried a portable oxygen canister when taken by a family member to shop or for any special outing. Dorris continued to bake delicious desserts and casseroles for family or church suppers, did the newspaper's daily jumble puzzle, read the *Charlotte Observer* every day, followed the news on television, and remained keenly interested in environmental, political, and other current issues. Knowing her lifelong wish, having been born only three years after the Nineteenth Amendment to the US Constitution was ratified, giving women the right to vote, I stood by her bedside two days before she died, and said, "Dorris, a woman is going to be president of the United States." Months later it was not to be, but in that moment we shared a sense of wonder and joy. Given the magnitude of the heartbreak she would have felt, for Dorris, the timing of her death may have been a blessing in disguise.

ADAPTING TO CHANGE

Being actively engaged in one's own life and in the lives of others is a vital factor in living well. So, too, is being open to and seeking change. If a person is planning to wait until 75 or 80 to learn to adapt to change, I would say, "Good luck with that!"

As we grow older across the long span of our lives, we become less similar to other people: The separate and unique cumulative experiences that shape our lifestyles and attitudes from our 20s into our 60s stand to shape how we will respond to the challenges of moving into our 70s, 80s, 90s, and beyond. "More than any other period in life, one enters old age with a past," write University of Michigan researchers Toni Antonucci and Hiroko Akiyama. "It is clear that some individuals have more and others fewer coping resources."[10]

In my mind, because you are the kind of person who would read a book like this, you're someone who values the lessons we can learn from other people in order to grow stronger, wiser, more flexible, and more able to embrace change. There is still time not to go into late adult life locked into inflexible attitudes and behaviors apt to make us less happy and our loved ones' lives more difficult.

Mary

Until she made the decision to "transition to something else but not yet retire," Mary served two decades as the much-beloved minister of a Presbyterian church in suburban Baltimore. At the age of 64, "I wanted to stay engaged and active, but gradually move into work that allows more time for family, especially my first grandchild." When sharing her views on "aging well," Mary knew exactly what she wanted to say.

"I'm very conscious now that I'm not going to the gym to have a movie star's body," she said, "but I try to keep my arteries clear and my body parts moving. I'm also trying to be more intentional about nurturing my relationships." Spending more time with loved ones has become a priority for Mary, probably to make up for the years when her ministry left too little quality time with family members and friends. As we age, "It will only get harder to become more flexible, more patient, and to exercise regularly, or lose weight—that won't *just* *happen*," she realizes. "A person has to grow into change."

Because her husband, Rocky, is 13 years older than she is, Mary thinks quite a lot about the likelihood of someday being alone again at the holidays: "Before, when I was divorced, my kids were little. Now they have their own families. What happens down the road when I wake up alone in the house? I'm going to have to let go of some of the habits, rituals, and traditions I value. We have to allow our children to have *their* rituals, and they'll be different."

Mary knows that "all families go through this as children become adults, especially those who live in the same town. So often everybody wants to claim them for the same time, at Christmas and Thanksgiving." Mary sees relinquishing family holidays (as they always were shared in the past) as "a growing edge for me, because I love being home and having everyone gathered around me. Already at Thanksgiving, we don't even try to get Rocky's daughters and their children. We have a brunch together with them on the Saturday after Thanksgiving." With Mary's daughter Rachel, son-in-law Matt, and their young son, who live in Virginia, five hours away, "We celebrated Christmas on January 17. It was fun!"

This year they will celebrate on Christmas night with her son David and his bride. "As time goes on," Mary explains, "it will only get harder to adapt and have things to look forward to. I can't control all aspects of aging, but I can work on becoming more flexible."

To Mary, aging well means that "we all have to look at what we can control and do those things in spades [to the greatest extent possible]. Aging and dying are part of the fabric of life. We need to face the anxiety, or we won't do right by our children or ourselves. I know my children love me and will be there to support me in whatever ways become necessary. But I must live *my* life so that they are free to live theirs. I want my family to be able to enjoy their lives to the fullest, and not feel they have to adjust their needs to fit my wants."

Knowing the family well, I'm sure Rachel and David will not let their mother be without their love and support in sickness, old age, or on her deathbed. Mary is confident that is true. At the same time, poets and psychologists alike say that loving our children means learning to release them. As Kahlil Gibran writes in *The Prophet*, "For life goes not backward nor tarries with yesterday. You are the bows from which your children as living arrows are sent forth."[11]

To Mary, to age gracefully is to focus on making our own lives meaningful: "Our gift to our adult children is seeing us involved and engaged in life—not waiting around for them to come visit us. I can't look to my kids to make me happy. I have to build a life that works for me. I hope I can say at 80 or 90 that I'm still living an interesting life."

THERE ARE MANY WAYS TO "RETIRE"— BE SURE TO CHOOSE THE RIGHT ONE FOR YOU

Mary is a good example of a person who sees her form of retirement as "a career change rather than a career exit," an opportunity to take on "new professional challenges and growth."[12] She is in the process of redesigning her work life to have more leisure time with her husband, adult children, new grandson, and old friends. She is planning to take a greater role in faith-based environmental work and advocacy. This has been a passion of Mary's, and she sees the environmental crisis, especially climate change, as an urgent moral issue. To Mary, working for a future in which the earth's resources are restored and protected not only builds on skills and insights she has developed through the years but is also the legacy she wishes to leave future generations. "I hope," Mary says, "that I can inspire my children and grandchildren to find their own ways of being involved in caring for the environment."

In a study published in March 2016, in the *Journal of Social Issues*, four researchers at the Yale School of Public Health found that people with positive retirement stereotypes of physical health and mental health in retirement *live longer* by 4.5 years and 2.5 years, respectively. Becca Levy and her colleagues, who "studied retirement stereotypes and survival over a 23-year period among 1,011 older adults," saw that people who think of retirement as a time of meaningfulness, activity, and growth "look forward to retirement as a new phase of life."[13]

The message here for all of us is clear: It is important to watch what we allow ourselves to believe about life as we grow older and older. If we expect to be lonely, immobile, sick, and dependent, that can become a self-fulfilling prophecy. While, once again, there are no guarantees, if we expect to be healthy, happy, involved, hopeful, active, independent, mobile, able, and satisfied in retirement, we have a far greater likelihood of living a meaningful and longer life.

"Sugar Man"

The husband of a friend of mine, known here as Sugar Man, was 66 when he retired after working 42 years as an iron and sheet metal worker for the Domino Sugar Plant. At a plant that processes 6.5 million pounds of sugar a day, he crafted, welded, installed, and repaired parts and equipment in every part of the refinery. It was dangerous work that often involved "pushing heavy welding machines, climbing a tall building, and sometimes working in 105–110 degree temperatures, so hot you couldn't put your bare hands on the railings," Sugar Man remembers. "They'd send four or five guys up there so we could rotate every 10 minutes. Several times I said, 'I'll work a few more minutes,' and I almost passed out."

There were also jobs that involved carrying a 50-pound cable on his shoulder while walking up a 50- or 80-foot ladder. "OSHA [Occupational Safety and Health Authority and Agency] said the electricians who change the light bulbs had to have a place to rest their backs every so many feet, or have a platform to stand on, on their way up to the [colossal red neon] Domino Sugars sign, atop the 12-story building, so we welded and installed the safety structures, all the way up. That place kept me in shape because I was always moving, but as the years went by there were aches and pains. Finally, the doctor said, 'You're wearing out your joints. When are you going to retire?'"

Sugar Man's wife encouraged her husband to retire. "I knew his work was hard, much of it outdoors," she told me. "Summers were brutal, winters were brutal. He could go on Social Security, collect a nice pension, and we wouldn't have to worry about him getting hurt."

He'll be 69 soon, and has been retired for nearly three years. "I can't believe how much I miss the people I worked with," Sugar Man says, "but not the job and the danger to my health. I still get up early, but I've moved it from 4:45 to 6:30 a.m. I do a five-mile walk three times a week, take my grandson to the school bus, and do chores around the house." A plumber and handyman, Sugar Man recently completely remodeled their kitchen—replacing the cabinets, counter tops, and appliances. His new hobby, shared with a son-in-law, is making his own beer. Sugar Man and his wife have also been able to travel, including to the Canadian Rockies and Yellowstone National Park. "She is great at arranging these trips, and we especially want to go back to Alaska," he tells me.

By far, the best part of his retirement is the quality time Sugar Man is sharing with grandson Aiden, who was 5 when his granddad retired, and is 8 years old now. "I was always working and didn't get to spend the time I wanted to spend with them when my daughters were growing up," Sugar Man says, wistfully. Perhaps that makes it all the sweeter to have these precious years with Aiden, at the school bus stop before and after school and when they hang out together at home. They especially enjoy going swimming and fishing together. "When I pass away, Aiden will always remember catching his first fish and his second fish with me," this grandfather realizes. "That first one was a five-pound bass, as big as any *I* ever caught, and Aiden said, 'Do you think my daddy will be proud of me?' I told him yes, and said *I'm* proud of you, too." Sugar Man wishes he could be as close to his other four grandchildren, who live several hours away. But, thanks to his having decided to retire at what turned out to be just the right time, he is able to look after Aiden when the boy's parents are at work, and his wife is free to drive to New Jersey nearly every week to help with their elder daughter's unexpected, newly born twins and the two older siblings.

"When I pass away," Sugar Man says for the second time—because it obviously means so much to him—"Aiden's not going to forget me." That is surely true. Having the gift of a loving, actively involved grandfather and all the good times they are sharing will always be a part of Aiden's fond memories and the formation of his character.

Jeannie

My former walking buddy, Jeannie, taught in a daylong kindergarten program, "until falling in love with these precious little children gave me a heartbreak every summer when I had to give them up." She then taught second grade, where "the best part of teaching continued to be nurturing the children, to help them become better people, which was more important to me than teaching them math," Jeannie explained. "But, of course, because they were nurtured, they did better with improving their academic skills anyway." After nearly 20 years, Jeannie left teaching. At the age of 50, "I didn't identify that as retiring," Jeannie told me, "because I was needed as a caregiver." Her mother had worsening Alzheimer's and needed frequent visits, and her daughter's best friend, and also her sisters, needed help with their new babies. When Jeannie's own grandchildren were born, she babysat them until the youngest was in school. She watched her cousin's grandkids for a few years after that. "*I always identified myself more as a caretaker than as a teacher, so after my parents died, and I wasn't babysitting anymore, that is when I had to adjust to retirement.*"

She is 67 now, walks often, runs occasionally, and tends her flower gardens to stay fit, and, joined by her best friend who is also her husband of 31 years, Jeannie enjoys family gatherings and regularly attending the grandsons' sporting, music, and other school events. No longer having the energy to take care of young children—but having found caregiving so meaningful, for virtually her entire adult life—Jeannie is finding that "it's hard to give up that sense of identity and purpose as a family caregiver." Because we all need to feel *needed and useful* in one way or another, and especially as we grow older, it's important to find new ways to live purposefully. Each of us in our own ways can offer small acts of kindness to others.

Lenny

For some people, retirement means "[putting] work-related identities permanently aside, while focusing on their connections to family, interests, and community activities," write research psychologists Kenneth Schulz and Mo Wang.[14] For my friend Lenny, working part time as the "marshal" for a public golf course is the perfect postretirement job. He rides around helping golfers, maintains their pace of play, and calms down the impatient, cranky ones who are waiting their turn to tee off on a lovely but busy day. For most of the 32 years during which he was passionately committed to opening doors of opportunity to students who might otherwise never have gone to college, Lenny reported to the president of a rapidly growing college. As the dean of students and director of enrollment development at Maryland's Anne Arundel Community College, his work was rewarding but highly stressful. Toward the end, "I had put on a lot of weight and didn't feel the same passion." By this time, Lenny had lost his younger sister, both of his parents, and his older brother, all within about seven years.

It was the death of his brother, at 59, that was the wake-up call. "He died of a heart attack," Lenny told me, "putting groceries in his car!" At 53, "I decided I was not going to die young and leave my family. My goal became retiring by the age Tony was when he died."

Not long before Lenny retired at 60, a member of the college's board of directors—seemingly out of the blue—asked Lenny, "Are you feeling alright? Make sure you take care of yourself. I'm worried about you. You look like you're under a lot of stress."

"During the first few months, I did consulting work that affirmed my decision to retire. I was very lucky to have been connected to people who trusted me, saw potential, and gave me opportunities. I got to do a job that I loved, work that was bigger than me, and inspired me—but I didn't want to do that anymore."

When Lenny went back to visit the college several years later, people said, "'You look fantastic! I can't believe how good you look.' I was doing photography, going birding, had lost a bunch of weight, was active, and eating right. I had an amazing sense of relief."

As a marshal on the golf course now, he is 68 years old. Lenny, who used to have a $20 million budget and 200 people under him, finds humor in the fact that, just sometimes, his job now is to handle conflict situations with guys belittling each other, trying to jump ahead of other players, and carrying on as if they're back in high school. "I almost quit a couple of times because of the confrontations I had to deal with," he says, "but you've got to let your ego go." On the golf course, "I get to talk to people, from 8-year-old kids to 90-year-olds still loving the game. I'm outdoors all day after three decades of working indoors. I watch the birds and the deer, and I get to hit balls at the practice range or play free rounds of golf anytime I'm not working."

In recent months, Lenny's wife had to have major surgery—brain surgery—followed by other hospital stays. She is recovering, but a long healing process is still underway. "I have so much respect for Judy and how she's handled it, how hard it is, and how well she has handled the pain and physical therapy," he says proudly. "We are closer than ever. My job recently has been to be here for my wife, to serve and support her. Getting her well and right again gives my life a lot of meaning."

Lenny says he feels "really grateful for the years of rewarding work" with students and a college president he was loyal to. "But now I just want to be the father of my kids, a good husband, and enjoy my grandkids." As far as aging goes, "I don't feel like we have to have a bucket list. It would be nice if we could do something like go back to Europe, but if we didn't get to do that, it wouldn't be a terrible thing. We have other things to do first. Being in the present is how I want to live."

Lenny says he does think about dying a lot and feels like he's running out of time. This is understandable since he came so close to losing Judy soon after the death of yet another sibling, leaving just three of the six of them still alive. "I do believe in God," he says. "This earth, this universe, is unbelievable, incomprehensible, magnificent. I see my grandchildren and they're magical. I'm just so thankful to have Judy."

Marian and Blake

For my friends since college Marian and Blake, both age 73, retirement links the past to the present. As Marian explains, "We are able to do many of the community service things we do *because* of what we learned in our professional lives." A PhD with a specialty in human factors (the field that designs technology so that it's easy to use), Blake left his management position at a major telecommunications company when continued downsizing made work less than enjoyable. Blake was 58 when he retired with a generous severance package. He had expected to do consulting work, but "after a short period of adjustment, I found that I liked not working," he recalls. Blake applies his intellect and skills to many volunteer activities. For six years, he served as the president and continues as a trustee of the Red Bank Chamber Music Society, an organization that sponsors five to seven professional concerts free and open to the community every year. For the River Rats, a local sailing club, Blake is a member of the board of trustees and teaches sailing classes to adults. He reads the *New York Times* every day, walks 18 to 30 miles weekly, lunches most weeks with a group of friends who call themselves the ROMEOs (retired old men eating out), works math problems for fun, and has built an awesome tree house for his grandchildren.

Marian retired twice. The first time was at age 56, from a high-stress corporate management position in health care. There was system-wide downsizing, and she could see that her own position was probably going to be affected within a year or two. She retired a second time at age 62 from her position as development / communications director for a regional Planned Parenthood affiliate. Within a year of her retirement, both of their sons were battling life-threatening illnesses, her mother's dementia was progressing to the point where her parents needed to be moved across the country to be closer to her brother, and Blake's only sibling was killed in a car accident! Marian is grateful that retirement allowed her to be fully available to her family, including traveling regularly between New Jersey and Minnesota to help care for her elderly parents for almost ten years.

Marian is a lifelong avid reader, belongs to a book club, enjoys museums, the theater, playing word and strategy games with family and friends, and doing volunteer work in her community. As a longtime member of the American Association of University Women, Marian takes special pleasure in fostering "equity for women and girls in a variety of ways." She participates in programs that teach salary negotiation skills to college students and leadership skills to high school girls, and supports experiences in science, technology, engineering, and math for middle school girls. Most recently, Marian and Blake have joined a group working to address climate change, work they hope will make a difference not just for their much-loved grandchildren but for those with whom they will share the future.

Looking back on those years of caregiving, Marian has a sense of gratitude. "I was able to help my parents when they most needed it, and I couldn't have done that as I did if I'd still been working, so I consider that a blessing of retirement," she says. "I have some painful memories from the last few years with my parents, but I also have happy ones that would never have occurred if I hadn't been with them. I'm grateful that they loved me for so long and so unconditionally. Having all those late years with my folks helped me make peace with the ways that they couldn't be what I wanted them to be when I was younger and was sometimes critical of them and their choices. Helping care for our parents further sealed the bonds between my brother and me; he was their faithful nearby caregiver, and it also gave me a chance to know my sister-in-law better. An especially sweet gift was to see my sons doing kind things for their grandparents."

Betty—94 Going on 95

At the round teak table in my dining room, we are 10, 20, and 30 years younger than Betty, but she bests us all in playing bridge. Since I'm the least skilled among the four of us, she wins more often when partnered with Val or Mary Jo. But Betty is very nice about it. "It's okay," she tells me graciously, "you're still learning." A smile comes over my face every time I think of her kind, re-assuring words of acceptance. To share good times with someone whose mind is sharp and whose personality is vibrant—a woman more than two decades ahead of me—truly does give me hope.

Born in 1921, Betty has suffered three enormous losses in her life, and yet she thrives today and is an upbeat, life-affirming, resilient person. I asked her, "How do you do it?" Before telling me how she dealt with tragedy while keeping her strong will to live, there is a background story Betty wanted me to know.

"I was a sturdy little girl with a mind of my own," she began. "I was high energy and my mother was not. She would say, 'Can't you ever be good?' Well, if 'being good' was sitting with my hands folded, that wasn't who I was. I ex-plored the neighborhood, even when I was young." She also survived scarlet fever, which had taken the life of her dad's little sister when she was only five. "I walked to school, home for lunch, and back to school—it was .7 miles—the first nine years, and it was a two-mile walk to and from high school."

Born to two college-educated parents, she finished college before marrying John, a recent graduate of MIT, who was an engineer like her father.

As a young couple, Betty and John played two-handed cards and Scrabble, and literally built their own house. "John would show me how to do things, and I mixed mortar until he finally got a cement mixer. I learned to glaze windows.

I put down tile in the bathroom while our first two children entertained themselves nearby. Merry was three and a half, and Steve was a year old. We kept him in the playpen while we worked."

Betty and John were still good together on the dance floor when celebrating their fiftieth wedding anniversary, surrounded by their extended family and many friends. Betty lost John three years later. That was 20 years ago. She speaks lovingly of her husband, without tears, grateful for their 53 years.

Understandably, Betty cries with continuing sorrow when she relives the story of losing Steven, their firstborn son. "He was an 18-year-old sophomore at the University of Pittsburgh, and had just been home for Christmas. It was snowing as I drove him to the Harrisburg airport. His little brother, Brad, was along to keep me company. I drove slowly to be safe, and we should have missed his plane, but we didn't. I wish so much that we had!"

On the way back to Baltimore, an announcement on the car radio reported that the plane had gone down in bad weather but that there were survivors. At home, Betty's husband heard the same news, was frantic, and called the airline desperate for information. After a long night of waiting, Alleghany Airlines called to say, "Your son is not identified among the living." One of Steven's professors called soon after, with condolences, to confirm that Steven had died.

Brad was 11, sister Cindy was 15, and Merry was 21. Everyone was devastated. "The plane crash was on Monday night," Betty continued. "When his body was brought back Thursday, I said, 'I don't think we should open the casket.' Later, the minister told us that was the right decision. There were just *remains*."

As would become a theme throughout Betty's life, she remembers being strengthened by the support they received: "People brought food, and so many friends reached out to us, from church and the neighborhood. The university sent a van filled with students to attend Steven's funeral." Then, and in the months and many years that followed, "I could always talk with my closest girlfriend, from church. People helped you go on with your activities." After reading in the newspaper that other college students had died in the crash, Betty and John corresponded with several of those bereaved parents. It was a way to mourn and find comfort together as the only other families who knew what it felt like to be them.

Something else in Betty's life and character that made her resilient is how she decided to respond to the terrible loss of losing Steven. *She wanted to protect her husband and surviving children from carrying an enduring, never-ending sorrow that would prevent them from ever being truly happy again.* "I felt very responsible to keep the family on an even keel," Betty explained. "I tried to get us back to normal living as soon as we could, to think about the living, and just appreciate all the love we had been shown."

Betty remembered how her paternal grandparents had responded to the loss of *their* son, her dad's brother, who died at the age of 21, from a rabid dog bite. "There was often sorrow in that house. As the first grandchild, I got to go there and spend the night, and I felt the sadness." Betty never knew the man who would have been her uncle, but she made an early decision based on observing her grandparents' sadness that seemed endless. Her grandparents used the money that was left in their young son's bank account to buy a beautiful brass clock, which they had placed on the mantle in their parlor to honor their son. "The clock bonged on the hour, and it reminded them constantly that their son was gone," Betty explained. "And I remember thinking at the time, that *I wouldn't do that.*"

Even as a young person Betty saw the contrast between her grandparents, who never stopped grieving, and her father. "My father survived losing his brother, and was a happy person who had sadness in his heart, but we could live a normal life. There was an example there for me."

She found a way to be a happy person. "I had to keep going, because we all shared this devastating loss of Steven, and we all had to keep going." Over time, Betty and her husband learned that some of their new friends had also lost children: one from a drunk driver, another from suicide, others from accidents. Betty and John talked with the other bereaved parents about a couple of valuable lessons they'd learned: "You don't get over it, but you can learn to live with it," and, "You can be an [uplifting] example to others—if you can keep going."

Betty and John did something that helped them mourn in a way they could manage, that may or may not help other bereaved parents: "We wanted to be around people who didn't know we'd lost a son, and we didn't tell them unless it developed one way or another." They took a free sailing course at a local high school, met a couple who had a boat, and went sailing on Maryland's Eastern Shore. Not so long after, Betty and John bought their own boat and joined a sailing club. "We made a lot of friends, became very competitive, raced our boat every Wednesday night, and even won beautiful trophies." For this couple, not having Steven's photo out in a prominent place in the house and spending time with new friends was how they could go on with their lives and feel strong enough to help their surviving children with their grief and healing process, too.

Betty's most recent journey through personal loss was her daughter Merry's nine-year battle with cancer and her death two years ago. Before Merry came close to the end, the family shared a wonderful cruise to the Caribbean—Betty, Merry and her husband, Dick, along with Merry's sister, Cindy, and their brother, Brad, and their spouses—all spending a week together, "where nobody had to cook." It was a way of cherishing the time each of them still had with Merry, and she with them. Near the end everyone gathered again, including Merry's three grown children and three granddaughters. "Merry had waited to get all those last hugs and kisses," Betty told me, "before she had the peaceful ending, and the death she might have chosen." Merry was 68 when she died.

The hardest part of Betty's long life is the loss of two children, her husband, two of her three siblings, and many friends. Betty, however, keeps making new friends, including me, and the women we get together with to play bridge, all of us considerably younger. "I'm not looking at age as a basis of friendship," she says. Betty's motto is, "Life is what happens to you while you are making other plans. The challenge we have is to accept this and move forward."

For the past six years, Betty has lived in a two-bedroom apartment at Oak Crest, a senior housing / multilevel-care community with several thousand residents and staff members. "I like my view," she says, appreciating the big windows in nearly every room. "I watch the sky all day, and the trees. Two Christmases ago, I asked for that chart in the kitchen that shows me all the different kinds of clouds."

Betty still drives her car short distances in daylight, navigates outings with a walker or cane, and gets around her own apartment without assistance. She is careful not to fall but remains active—cooking her own breakfast and lunch, playing bridge twice a week, attending religious services, eating every Tuesday night with her friend Susie, and always going downstairs for her early evening meal. Once a month, Merry's husband, Dick, comes to visit and they go to dinner together. Her grandson, Randy, lives about 30 minutes away, and sometimes Betty has him over to play a peg board game. Betty also likes to read, faithfully watches the news and the Baltimore Orioles baseball games on TV, and stays in touch with her family mostly by telephone. Her son, Brad, manages Betty's finances from his home in Florida and calls her every Sunday night.

"I think my 'kids' appreciate that I'm self-sufficient," Betty says. "There is nothing worse than a sour old person."

When I asked Betty if it took some time for her to adjust when she sold her home and moved to independent living at Oak Crest Village, she replied, "Well, some people complain all the time and it doesn't do any good. I'm a happy person."

There was one more thing. A friend who knows that Betty was born and reared in Massachusetts has an explanation for Betty's strength and unbroken spirit. "She says," Betty tells me proudly, "It's my New England backbone!"

A "CONVOY" OF SUPPORTIVE PEOPLE

Author Laura E. Berk, in *Development Through the Lifespan*, asks her readers to visualize a convoy of ships to understand the network of relationships that protect and support us during our life's journey. The ships surrounding ours, sailing alongside, are our closest family members and friends. "Those less close, but still important, travel on the outside," she says. "With age, ships exchange places in the convoy, and some drift off while others join in the procession. As long as the convoy continues to exist, [we] adapt positively."

In the years after losing their eldest son, Betty and John were literally protected and helped to move through their troubled waters by a convoy of "ships"—the sailboats, and the new friends who sailed them—enabling these bereaved parents to absorb their loss gradually, at their own pace, and in a safe environment. Displayed on a shelf in her independent living apartment, reminding Betty of the strong support system that included her husband, John, and their sailing friends, are seven beautifully crafted trophies, model sailboats made from a combination of exotic wood from teak, cherry, mahogany, cedar, and walnut trees. Betty continues to thrive in her "old age" by staying in contact with family, making new friends, and keeping the old ones as long as possible.

Studies in the United States, Canada, Israel, Japan, Germany, and France have examined the impact of social relationships on mental health. While experts disagree somewhat in their findings as to *how many* people are needed in our support system—our "convoy of ships"—what affects our health and sense of well-being in favorable or unfavorable ways is the *quality* of our relationships. Although "the majority of relationships include at least a little negativity and/or conflict," as Toni Antonucci and her research colleagues report, the people in some of those ships do more harm than good! The best way to "cope with specific stressful life events and daily hassles"[15] is to maximize your time with positive people and minimize your time with negative people.

If someone in your "convoy" frequently gives "unasked for support and unsolicited advice," leaving you to feel incompetent, or "behaves badly" by withholding love and affection, or engages in "more direct and purposefully hurtful behaviors, such as hostility and dismissiveness," as Antonucci describes it, *severely limit your time with that person!* Such negativity can increase your health risks and even affect your mortality. To protect your psychological and physical health, and to increase your life satisfaction and happiness, what is needed from the people in your support system is trust, reassurance, and respect.

In my 40 years as a psychologist, the scientific evidence has grown stronger and stronger demonstrating that our mental and physical health—*and our longevity*—are inextricably tied to the love, caring, and support we exchange with the people who matter in our lives.

Making Life Easier for Those Who Someday Will Take Care of You

Making lives meaningful in old age is new. It therefore requires more imagination and invention than making lives merely safe does.
—Atul Gawande, MD

Sooner rather than later, it is important—for all of us—to have honest and on-going conversations with our spouse, adult children, or any other person on whom we will need to rely in sickness, disability, or old age. There are legal documents we need to have in place to protect our loved ones and ourselves. There are quality of life issues critical to discuss *before* we become physically or cognitively impaired enough to need help to manage our daily lives. There are medical documents and directives needed to help guide our family members in making decisions with our physicians. In addition, as odd as it may seem that this needs emphasis, we need to help our loved ones get to *know* us better! In order to make *their* lives easier as our future caregivers and *our* lives worth living, as long as possible, we need to share more specifics about the cherished experiences, challenges, accomplishments, and simple pleasures of our lives thus far. What experiences, what things, large and small, have we valued and found meaningful?

"HABITS OF A LIFETIME"

In her helpful book of advice for caregivers, *Creating Moments of Joy*, Jolene Brackey devotes a chapter to "habits of a lifetime." If, one day, it happens that the ability to communicate is lost, even temporarily, loved ones and other caregivers need to know "the important details of a person's history, passions, and interests" in order to help him or her overcome daily struggles, Brackey explains. She emphasizes that wants and wishes must be known ahead of time, as illustrated well in the story she tells about a retired Texas Ranger. Imagine that the man described below is *your beloved uncle*, being cared for in an assisted living facility where the staff members don't *know* him, and the message of the story will be soon evident:

> The staff told me about a belligerent man who was still [able to function mentally] but very uncooperative. I knocked on his door and walked into his room about 9:00 at night. The room was very warm, he was resting on top of his covers with his day clothes on, and there were pictures of horses all over his room. I explained I was just visiting and asked him about the pictures of horses on the wall. He eagerly told me how he was a Texas Ranger and rode all over the United States to compete in rodeos. We had a delightful conversation about him sleeping under the stars and being a bachelor all of his life roaming the countryside. When I left the room I thought about our conversation. He sleeps on top of the covers with his clothes on because he is accustomed to sleeping under the stars, and his room is really warm because he is used to the heat living in Texas. If he did not have pictures of horses around him, he would essentially lose his sense of identity. With this new information, I was able to understand him. Can you tell me why he was "uncooperative"? He's never been married. Now he has 30 women telling him what to do. Instead of labeling him, the staff should have seen this as an opportunity to write down his habits of a lifetime while he is still able to communicate. Imagine how aggressive he would be if he had Alzheimer's and we tried to put him in pajamas and tuck him into bed.[1]

Jolene Brackey has it right: "We are all just around the corner, or maybe a few corners, from needing someone to care for us. If you write down your habits of a lifetime you are more likely to get the kind of care you want and need."[2] Consider this question: How can our loved ones interact with us meaningfully, provide us with the simple pleasures we increasingly value in disability or old age, or make consequential decisions related to our care if we aren't *known* to them?

Here are some questions you can answer in a journal or letter or (better yet) talk about in person with your loved ones, asking them to do the same with you: What jobs have you had in your life? What skills were learned? Who are the people you've helped? What are some of the challenges you've overcome? What are some of your accomplishments? Growing up, who were the people who influenced you? In what ways did they impact your life for good? What experiences shaped your beliefs and values? What activities (games, sports, music, subjects in school, travel, or pets) did you most enjoy? Which of these things do you still find fun or fulfilling? What kind of music comforts or uplifts you? Which outdoor activities, favorite foods, TV shows, topics of discussion, and simple pleasures have meant something to you during your lifetime and lift your spirits still?

MY NEIGHBOR

It is a hot and ridiculously muggy mid-July day in Baltimore. I don't even walk our dog on a miserable day like this, but I see my 90-year-old neighbor near the small lake across the street, pushing a yellow lawn mower that is twice the size of any I've ever seen. Although it is theoretically self-propelled, he is having to maneuver it by physical force, repeatedly lifting the heavy thing as he mows around the four corners of 20 or more wooden roadside posts. Watching from my driveway, seeing him sweating profusely and hatless, I try to think who could come do the work instead. This is a really nice man—my neighbor for the last 35 years—and I'm afraid he's going to keel over right in front of me. He shuts down the machine when I walk over and says, "I *like* the heat. My mowing man says it's too hot for him, and has been promising to come for two weeks." I ask my neighbor to come inside for a glass of water, into air conditioning, and we sit for a while in my kitchen. While our poor walk-deprived border collie licks my neighbor's hands and knees, I mention this book I'm writing, and he tells me his story.

My neighbor lives alone in a big house on his four-acre property. He is a semiretired certified public accountant whose company, passed down from his father, continues in business. He doesn't go into the office anymore, but "they give me software on my computer to do tax returns for family members," he says.

He met his wife of 62 years on a tennis court when they were both 14, loved her dearly, and thinks of her every day. After she passed away five years ago, he missed her terribly and got online to find a companion. "The dating site sent me volunteers who were the age of my children. *I didn't want children.*

So a friend of mine got me on a different dating site and I found this woman whose first husband was a lawyer and second husband was a doctor. When you meet people this way, you expect them to be treasure seekers, but she's wealthier than I am. On her ninetieth birthday, she took her friends and family on a cruise and we shared a room. The family wanted me to make a speech about our relationship, so this is what I said":

> Visualize a 1,000-piece puzzle. You dump the box on the floor, and you randomly pick two pieces up, entirely different on top, strangely shaped. You place them together, and they're a perfect fit.

When they first met online four years ago, my neighbor explained, "She said, 'I'm liberal, I'm Jewish.' And I said, 'I'm liberal. I'm nothing.' We love each other and we talk about our ex-spouses over and over again. Both families are very happy for us. She's 92 now."

His companion lives in a nursing home and uses a walker more often now. He drives himself to have dinner with her three nights a week (where gentlemen must wear jackets), sleeps over two of those nights, and they enjoy a special speaker at her facility every Wednesday evening. My neighbor is the kind of person whose energy and contentment with his life make you smile listening to him talk, because there's a wry sense of humor breaking through nearly every subject. "She always dresses immaculately and goes to the hairdresser," he says. "I don't wear green, blue, and yellow all together anymore. I had her write on a piece of paper a list of two colors that go together, put it on my closet door, and I read this thing to put my clothes on."

They go to the symphony and to their favorite restaurants, watch movies at his house, and often take classes at a local church that are offered by Odyssey, the lifelong learning program of Johns Hopkins University. In one of the classes, they took a field trip to visit the US Supreme Court, and in another a physics professor lectured on the subject of time, explaining what Einstein figured out before anyone else.

When I ask to what he attributes his long and "damn good life so far," my neighbor replies, "Three things. Be very lucky. Be born recently enough to have your life saved, throughout your life, by medicines and new medical techniques. And, every time something bad happened to me something good happened, too." He was 17, during World War II, when he started college at Johns Hopkins University and became a platoon leader in the ROTC, a college leadership program for the army. "By the time the invasion of Europe had started from Great Britain, they kept testing me," he recalls. "I had turned 18, was in the infantry, they tested me some more, and—just before I would have gone to Europe for the Battle of the Bulge, when the Germans had almost turned things around—they sent me to Yale to learn Japanese. I was put in the counterintelligence corps and sent to Japan the minute the war was over. By then I had amassed the speaking capabilities of a 5-year-old Japanese boy, but I teamed up with a Hawaiian and together we did alright. We were interrogating soldiers, trying to find out if they served where the worst atrocities took place."

My neighbor is "still having fun," he says. His daughter Peggy lives locally and visits regularly, "but she would be happier if I'd go live in a retirement home, in case I get dementia later on, and they might not take me." His sons come from out of state, along with their spouses, to visit for a month every year. He is happy living in his own house. "I scurry a lot," he says, tending his property; "I walk a mile a couple of days a week, and swim two or three times a week." Does he swim laps in his own pool? I ask. "No, I just lie on my back and look at the sky."

His doctor says, "You're in magnificent condition, but I can't guarantee that you aren't going to have a stroke."

My neighbor, however, hopes to live and die right where he is. With exuberance he adds, "I just got a drone for fun! My daughter Peggy has a farm and I can fly it there."

ATTENTION FAMILY MEMBERS: MOST FOLKS *DON'T* GET DEMENTIA!

"Severe memory loss is *never* a normal part of growing older," explain Nancy Mace and Peter Rabins, in *The 36-Hour Day*, a book newly updated and widely recognized as the definitive guide for families caring for a loved one with dementia. "According to the best studies available, 8 to 10 percent of older people have a severe intellectual impairment, and 10 to 15 percent may have milder impairments. The diseases that cause dementia become more prevalent in people who survive into their 80s and 90s, but 50 to 70 percent of those who live to age 90 never experience a significant memory loss or other symptoms of dementia. Difficulty recalling names or words is common as we age but usually is not enough to interfere with our lives."[3]

Treatable Diseases or Conditions That Mimic Dementia

Singer and songwriter Kris Kristofferson, age 80, was misdiagnosed as having Alzheimer's disease. He suffered a significant cognitive decline, was depressed, and took the wrong medicines *for three years* before being diagnosed with Lyme disease (an infection that typically occurs several weeks or even months after a deer tick bite). An attending physician at Harvard Medical School and an expert in the treatment of tick-borne illnesses, Dr. Nevena Zubcevic told a group of Martha's Vineyard Hospital physicians in 2016 that Kristofferson was "cured of dementia" once his Lyme disease was treated by one of the many doctors he consulted. In her urgent reminder to other physicians, Zubcevic described Lyme disease as widespread and frequently overlooked: "The bull's-eye rash only happens 20 percent of the time, and [the tick wound] can often look like a spider bite or a bruise," she said. "*Sudden-onset dementia should really be a red flag for Lyme, especially in people with compromised immune systems. Everyone over 50 has a compromised immune system.*"[4]

Kristofferson's wife told the *Huffington Post*, "There is not that big black void ahead of us anymore. He is so much better now than he was three years ago." Kristofferson has even started scheduling concerts again.[5]

Some of the other "treatable conditions that mimic dementia," were named by Margery Rosen in a recent *AARP Bulletin*: (1) *Normal pressure hydrocephalus*, which is usually first noticed when the person has a slow shuffle gait and walks with his or her legs spread wide apart for balance. Some accompanying symptoms are memory and thinking problems, urinary incontinence, or a frequent need to urinate. (2) *The side effects of medications and the drug interactions of multiple medicines* also can produce symptoms similar to the memory problems seen in dementia, plus confusion, paranoia, and aggression. (3) *A vitamin B12 deficiency*, known as *pernicious anemia*, can cause "nerve damage such as numbness or tingling in the hands and feet, confusion, personality changes, irritability, depression, and forgetfulness." (4) *A urinary tract infection* can cause "memory problems, confusion, delirium, dizziness, agitation, even hallucinations," explains Rosen. "UTIs are often missed in older people because seniors rarely have the typical symptoms of a high fever or pain." (5) *A thyroid problem* "may trigger dementia-like symptoms," such as forgetfulness, fatigue, depression, and anxiety, yet be "mistaken for normal aging" because the disorder develops over time, and half of the "roughly 30 million people (most over age 50) who have thyroid disease ... don't even know it." (6) *Diabetes* "damages blood vessels in the brain" and can result in "memory problems, confusion, irritability, [and] inattention"—*if not caught early or prevented in the first place.* (7) "*Alcohol abuse* . . . destroys brain cells in the areas critical for memory, thinking, decision making, and balance," but "depending on the damage, the effects of long-term alcohol abuse can sometimes be reversed."[6]

Depression is another condition that can mimic dementia (listed by Rosen in the *AARP Bulletin* referenced above), but it is a subject worth discussing separately. The relationship between depression and dementia is complex because cognitive impairments such as poor concentration, difficulty in making decisions, and muddled thinking can be mistakenly diagnosed as dementia, instead of being recognized a treatable depression. In the words of Hai Kang, Ravi Prakash, and their team of researchers from China, Italy, and India, "The timely recognition and treatment of depression in the elderly is thus important not only to prevent the patient from the consequences of progressing depression but also to prevent [him or her] from unnecessary investigative evaluations for dementia." What can make an accurate diagnosis difficult "arises from the two facts that cognitive impairments can be found in depression and that dementia can manifest with depressive symptoms as well."[7]

According to the Centers for Disease Control and Prevention, "The good news is that the majority of older adults are *not* depressed. Some estimates of major depression in older people living in the community range from less than 1% to about 5% but rise to 13.5% in those who require home healthcare and to 11.5% in older hospital patients."[8] The problem, however, explains physician Walter A. Brown, is "that between 20 percent and 40 percent of patients with dementia also suffer major depression and that up to 70 percent have some depressive symptoms. This depression warrants and responds to treatment." Brown adds that "depression may place people at increased risk for dementia or may be an early manifestation of dementia."[9]

Polypharmacy, defined as "the use of multiple prescription drugs or more medicines than are medically necessary,"[10] can lead to clouded thinking, paranoia, memory and other cognitive problems, impairments in day-to-day self-care and functioning, and increase the risk of adverse drug interactions and falls! In an 11-year national study, "outpatients taking five or more medications had an 88 percent increased risk of experiencing an Adverse Drug Event (ADE) compared to those who were taking fewer medications." In two other studies, the rate of ADEs among nursing home residents was "twice as high in patients taking nine or more medications compared to those taking less," and older military veterans "taking more than five medications [were] almost four times as likely to be hospitalized from an Adverse Drug Event. As one might expect, common drug classes associated with ADEs include anticoagulants, NSAIDs, cardiovascular medications, diuretics, antibiotics, anticonvulsants, benzodiazepines, and hypoglycemic medications."[11] Another problem is the overuse among people with dementia of antipsychotic medications—drugs which are frequently unnecessary or used at higher doses and much longer than necessary, and far too often make the person with dementia *more* confused or agitated.

The best ways to stop or improve the problems of polypharmacy are (1) *to carry in one's wallet a current list of every drug, over-the-counter medicine, and vitamin supplement* being taken, to copy for each doctor who has any contact with you or your loved one; (2) to *have all prescriptions filled at the same pharmacy*, where possible drug interactions will pop up on the pharmacist's computer screen; (3) to ask the elderly person's physician, when there is any reason for concern, to *work as a team with a clinical pharmacist*; and (4) to *ask for informed consent to be obtained before there is any use of antipsychotic medications*, and for antipsychotics to be used only in accordance with the American Psychiatric Association's (updated and revised) May 2016 guidelines: limited use of antipsychotics, "only employing them when agitation or psychosis is severe, nondrug interventions have been tried first, risks are discussed with the patient or surrogate decision maker, dosage is begun at a minimum level and tapered *off if there is 'no significant response' after four weeks.*"[12]

For all of the above reasons, it is very important for older persons with any worrisome cognitive impairments to be followed regularly by their family doctor, but also to be evaluated by a geriatrician (a physician who has completed a residency in either internal medicine or family medicine plus a fellowship in the medical, social, and psychological issues that concern older adults). If you don't have access to a geriatrician, consider getting a second opinion from another practitioner if your doctor is unresponsive to questions about medications or other kinds of care. Anyone who is depressed needs to be evaluated and treated by a psychiatrist, a geriatrician, or another physician with expertise in treating depression in the elderly.

IF HELP IS NEEDED—AT HOME OR IN A FACILITY— HERE'S WHAT YOUR LOVED ONES NEED TO KNOW

We all can only do whatever is the best we can do at the time. Sometimes all of the choices we have are undesirable, may carry a burden of regret, but are necessary for financial, medical, or other reasons including the caregiver's mental health and well-being. Before our decisions are made, however, we should ask whether there aren't some wise and welcome choices that we're unaware of—because of how we think about our options, or unknowingly limit ourselves from a lack of information, or because we're not seeing the big picture. Throughout my adult life, I've been struck by how profoundly our decisions, and the quality of our lives, can change for the better with the benefit of a new perspective. If we're open to new knowledge, we can plan for the challenges ahead.

Many assisted living facilities and nursing homes are marketed with "visuals" designed to impress the children of older people with their attractive hotel-like features yet lack the ratio of staff to residents needed to help elders remain as mobile and active as possible. These beautiful and safe environments, stresses physician Atul Gawande, appeal to the family members making decisions for their loved one but "almost never sell themselves as places that put a person's choices about how he or she wants to live first and foremost."[13]

There are a number of reasons why it is not a good idea to leave this decision making entirely to our loved ones or wait until the need is great to discuss options and priorities for our own elder care. In Gawande's best-selling book, *Mortal Lives*, he quotes assisted living expert Keren Brown Wilson's insights:

> It's the rare child who is able to think, "Is this place what Mom would want or like or need?" It's more like they're seeing it through their own lens. The child asks, "Is this a place I would be comfortable leaving Mom?"
>
> Assisted living isn't really built for the sake of older people so much as for the sake of their children . . . They tout their computer lab, exercise center, and their trips to concerts and museums—features that speak more to what a middle-aged person desires for a parent than to what the parent does. Above all, they sell themselves as safe places.
>
> We want autonomy for ourselves and safety for those we love . . . Many of the things we want for those we care about are things that we would adamantly oppose for ourselves because they would infringe upon our sense of self.[14]

There are surely times when an elderly person is so profoundly debilitated that a nursing home is necessary. Sometimes, simply no other care is available or affordable. At other times, "out of love and devotion," family members may *think* they have "no choice" but to put their elderly loved one in the very place their loved one has long dreaded: a nursing home, "with people in their wheel-chairs all slumped over and lined up in corridors," or a place where one's life is "reduced to a bed, a dresser, a tiny TV, and half of a room with the curtain between him and someone else." Asks Gawande, "Why?"

If a person is like my still-active and clear-thinking 90-year-old neighbor, or even an elderly person with significant impairments but who has "a friend, a routine, some things he still [likes] to do," why not let him stay where he is? If choosing between being safer in a nursing home or being happier where he might suffer a fall, and die before someone found him in time, it's likely that "he'd choose the happier place. So why choose differently?"[15]

Here's part of what I will tell my own daughters. Plan A: "If it is in any way possible, please let me stay in my own home, or live independently in an apart-ment near your home, with reasonable accommodations made for safety's sake or disability. If needed, get outside help from a reputable nursing agency or through a careful hiring process, so that I can have the quality care described below, and so *you're* not burdened." Plan B: "If necessary, or it turns out that there is a facility where the residents are treated as described below, and if there are meaningful activities for me to enjoy that include outings with others and with you, *that* will be alright, too. Of course, dear daughters, if you can, please visit me often—enough to monitor that the caregiving is kind and respectful, while keeping me active and mobile—and to give me the pleasure of your com-panionship, conversations with news of your lives, and your wonderful hugs and kisses. If you have career or family obligations that take you far away from where I am, please find a trusted person nearby who can visit with me and see that I am being cared for in a warm and respectful way, and visit with me via Skype or other electronic means until you can visit in person."

It's Not Only the Place but How a Person Is Treated

Yes, you might want to tell your family members—if you feel this way—that there are things worse than having a fall, stroke, or heart attack and dying alone in your own home. At the same time, here's what you will want your spouse, adult children, or other loved ones to remember if one or more of them provide your care as you grow older, if it becomes necessary for you to have nursing care at home, or they are choosing a senior housing, assisted living, or nursing facility:

- *People in the least dignified and most dependent situations desperately need respect, courtesy, and patience from their caregivers.* As a family member, you'll want to pay close attention to the way *you* speak and also how your in-home or facility caregivers talk to your loved one. Notice if caregivers use controlling language: words like "must," or "ought," or talk down to your elderly person as if he or she is a child (or a puppy!) in a sing-song voice, or scold him or her. Caregivers should not call the person old enough to be their mother or grandfather by demeaning pet names like "dearie" or "honey," or by his or her first name instead of "Miss Jane," or "Dr. Ann," or "Mr. Jones," unless that is the care receiver's preference.

- *Caregivers who give explanations, offer choices, give feedback, and use words of courtesy or encouragement communicate respect and promote self-respect in the person dependent on their care*: "Here's what I'm going to do next . . ." "Do you want this one or that one?" "I think you look nice in that color." "Please," and "Thank you," are also ways of speaking that affirm the dignity of your loved one.

- *Elders who are impaired need extra time to do the things for themselves they're still able to do.* Plenty of additional time is needed for bathing or dressing when there's someplace to go (bathroom, dinner, religious service, ride in the car, doctor's visit). Nonprofit facilities tend to have more caregivers on staff per resident, which allows for individualized care. Caregivers should be *person centered* instead of *task centered*. Promoting autonomy and independence will help maintain the elder person's level of ability, instead of treating him or her as a passive object on an assembly line of tasks to complete.

- Everyone needs and appreciates genuine compliments, particularly in late adulthood when many activities of daily living become harder to do. *If the praise being given or the attention being shown to your loved one by the caregiver seems overdone, showy, or inauthentic, however, you justifiably may wonder whether what you are seeing is not how your loved one is being treated when you aren't there!* You will want to observe more often and more carefully the caregiver's behavior and your elderly loved one's reactions to him or her. (What psychologists call "reaction formation" is an insincere, overdone, extravagant expression of positive emotion that masks one's negative feelings.) Does the caregiver go on and on—in a way that seems insincere—about how they "just *love*" taking care of your father, or think your mother is "the most *wonderful* person ever," *while you are seeing mood changes or getting other nonverbal messages from your parent that this caregiver is someone he or she really doesn't like?* The Shakespearian version of this phenomenon is "the lady doth protest too much, methinks," meaning that a person trying so hard to convince you of their loyalty and good will may in fact be someone you are wise *not* to trust.

- *It is also essential that caregivers respect the care recipient's cultural and religious beliefs (or lack thereof) and not impose their own religious beliefs and practices.*

- *Quality of life matters! Pleasurable experiences, meaningful throughout our lifetimes, are still possible even when a person has dementia.* "Researchers have observed," write Nancy Mace and Peter Rabins, in *The 36-Hour Day*, "that people who had previously paced, screamed, and struck out became relaxed and had fewer distressing and disruptive behaviors when they participated in enjoyable activities."[16]

- *Reciprocity matters.* We spend our entire lives talking back and forth with each other. A person with dementia (just as in a coma or in hospice care) needs to hear others speak about their own lives in a sharing and conversational way ("let me tell you about what your granddaughter did today . . ."), as well as to hear an ongoing affirmation of who they were and are ("what I respect and love about you is . . .").

Sexual Activity at Any Age

For many, one of the most difficult topics to discuss is sexuality . . . especially with our children. But we do not cease to be sexual beings as we age, although sexual expression may take new forms. As you think about your own aging process and discuss it with your loved ones, it is often helpful to be aware of how aging and sexuality are not mutually exclusive.

- *"Don't try to convince yourself that sex isn't important,"* advises psychologist and couples therapist Susan Fletcher, writing in the May 2016 issue of the *AARP Bulletin*. "A man trying to deal with his wife's low sexual desire, for example, tells himself it's not important so he won't feel rejected. Then he loses the real emotional connection."[17]

- In nursing homes, "Flirting is a common and socially acceptable behavior for men and women," write gerontology experts Mace and Rabins. "It makes a person feel younger and more attractive." As for the idea that inappropriate sexual behavior is associated with senility, "There is *no* basis to this myth," emphasize Mace and Rabins: "Inappropriate sexual behaviors in people with illnesses that cause dementia are uncommon" and very rare. "Occasionally a father may make inappropriate advances to his daughter. *This is not incestuous behavior.* While it can be terribly upsetting for everyone, it usually means only that he is unable to recognize familiar people . . . Daughters often look much like their mothers did when the mother was a young wife . . . Gently redirect him when this happens, and try not to be too distressed."[18]

- And if someone is masturbating, he or she "is only doing what feels good." This is not a problem if the person is alone and others ignore it, or if family members or staff react in a matter-of-fact fashion and lead the person to a private place. Aimless self-touching or itching in the genital area may signal a urinary tract infection, which should be checked out by a physician.[19]

A 93-year-old widower told me that he "had the operation" 20 years ago, where an erection is not possible, "but who cares? Why would anybody think sex was bad? Why isn't it great?" Referring to his relationship over the past several years with his 91-year-old companion, the retired college teacher added, "She told me she hadn't had sex in four or five years, and I'm trying to remedy that. Last night she said it was the best she'd ever had!" As it happens, he said, "Today, in the *New York Times*," there is a feature story, "Too Old for Sex? Not at This Nursing Home." He has already clipped it out for his lady. Later, I will read this article by Winnie Hu: it's all about the Hebrew Home in Riverdale, the Bronx, a facility that has a "sexual expression policy" to allow residents to have intimate, consensual relationships in privacy.[20] Of the 870 seniors in this nursing home, about 40 are in a relationship. Wrapping up this happy topic, the widower declares, "Thank God for women!"

"BE LIKE THE SUN"

Human nature being what it is, the more you try to coerce someone into doing something, the more apt they are to resist. To illustrate this very human trait of resistance to coercion, Jolene Brackey uses the analogy of "a sun and a cloud fighting over who was the most powerful and the strongest." Seeing a little boy down below, explains Brackey, the sun and the cloud agreed that "whoever gets that jacket off the little boy wins." First, the cloud floated over to the boy and—with its blowing wind—it blew and blew, until its energy was spent. "What did the little boy do? He held on even tighter to his jacket." Having tried and tried to the point of exhaustion, the cloud gave the task over to the sun. "The sun didn't move. He just waited and warmed up. He radiated his warmth. He was very patient. The little boy started to sweat . . . [and] took off his jacket." The moral of the story, continues Brackey, is that caregivers who are "more like the sun and radiate warmth" are more likely to receive a cooperative response. Especially when warmth and patience are accompanied with an understandable explanation, the person receiving the care is less apt to resist a family member or employed caregiver's requests.[21]

Not only can we ask our loved ones to "be like the sun" when our turn comes to be the person cared for, we can also ask our family members to "live in our truth." As discussed in chapter 9, it is not lying but meeting a person where they are to make up an answer ("he's still at work") when your parent with advanced Alzheimer's is looking around the house for her long-deceased husband. "A person wouldn't ask these questions," writes Brackey, "unless it is very real in her mind. This is her truth and we need to live in her truth. Guess who has to change. You do! They are doing the best they can with the abilities they have left. So do all you can do to make whatever or whomever they are looking for seem perfectly OK."[22]

How our family members and any paid caregivers in the future communicate with us in disability or old age will make all the difference in the quality of our lives. Brackey emphasizes wise thinking, compassion, and kindness—especially when cognitive impairments cause anxiety and distress: "People with dementia can hear, think, and feel emotions! Do not talk over, through, or about them as if they are not there. Avoid whispering because it arouses suspicion. Yelling into a person's ear who cannot hear very well will only upset or frighten them."[23] All of these insights and words of advice will apply equally well, whether in our old age we have dementia or are just slowing down with some other impairments.

GERALD: STILL THRIVING BUT PLANNING AHEAD

He is 84, an amazingly strong fellow both physically and spiritually. I first met Gerald and his wife, Eileen, in a water aerobics class at our community pool.

They have three daughters, six grandkids, and a step-granddaughter. Eileen is an RN who taught student nurses until she retired 12 years ago, at age 67, "to become a full-time grandmother."

Years ago, the couple lost two babies born prematurely. They also suffered the devastating loss of Michael, their 13-year-old son, following his three-year battle with leukemia. "Loss either tears you apart or draws you closer," Eileen says. "I thought I would die, and it would have been easier if I *had* died instead of Michael, but I got through my time of questioning God because of Gerald's unfaltering faith. Gerald helped me believe that the Lord saw the whole picture, that our lives were and are in God's hands."

After serving as a radio operator in the US Navy, Gerald had graduated in industrial education from the University of Maryland. He worked for Bendix, then Westinghouse, where "he was a wonderful writer, with a gift for words and grammar," according to his wife. His job involved writing manuals to explain how to operate and maintain all sorts of equipment, big and small, produced by the plants. "We were blessed," Eileen explained, "that, before being laid off, Gerald had just enough time with Westinghouse to get a partial pension and medical benefits." He was 58, started substitute teaching, and began a long career of doing handyman jobs. "Gerald's mom died when he was 12, and when he lost his dad at 17," Eileen went on, "he learned plumbing and electrical work from my dad, who treated him like a son. So he can fix practically anything."

Gerald was an elder in the church until the age of 70, Eileen continued, clearly proud of her husband of 58 years. He helped with Communion, visited the sick, and taught Sunday school. After more than 20 years, he still works the polls at election time. "Gerald has a gentle disposition, an inquiring mind, is the most even-tempered person in the world, and loves people," Eileen told me. Even with a considerable bend in his back these days, at 84, he continues to help "older people" around the neighborhood with weeding and hedge trimming. Their daughter, who is a teacher and "can use the money in the summer," takes guidance from her dad and does more and more of the work with him.

Gerald and Eileen have fond memories of taking trips to Disney World when their children were young, sightseeing and camping in national parks in the western United States, and taking their pop-up trailer across Canada. Ten or 15 years ago, the couple enjoyed a cruise through the Panama Canal and to a number of Caribbean islands. Their married life is enriched most of all by the time they spend transporting their grandchildren to school and swimming events, feeding them at their home while the parents are at work, and spending time together with their three daughters and extended family. Eileen swims laps in the community pool, and they are regulars in the water aerobics class where Eileen exercises and Gerald mostly likes to float around and talk to everyone while they exercise.

What they are doing to make life easier for their children as they continue to age includes "clearing out stuff we don't need in the house, so if we have to move our daughters won't have to deal with that." They also have a will and the other needed documents listing each daughter in succession as their durable power of attorney and medical power of attorney. (See appendix C.) "Our advance medical directive," Eileen explains, "states that—if a doctor and our daughter who is a nurse practitioner agree that there is no hope—we do not want any heroics. If prolonging the inevitable, there's no point. Let the Lord do his will. He had us in His care before we were born."

PROTECTING OUR LOVED ONES
AND HELPING THEM PROTECT US

When my parents were getting frail but still living in their own Oklahoma home, my sister, brother, and I lived in Texas, Oregon, and Maryland. We arranged for our folks to have Meals on Wheels delivered every weekday, and we hired a daytime companion who also did light housekeeping for them. My older sister and brother, both retired, visited them often and would stay two or more weeks at a time, while my young daughters and I visited twice a year. At one point, we siblings became concerned that a neighborhood lady, who'd been "volunteering" as a helper to our parents, might be trying to get my father to change his will and include her! We were relieved to learn from our parents' lawyer in another city that our parents' separate revocable living trusts (held by the attorney) were providing our mother and father with legal protections from interference with their estate planning.

My parents had protected themselves—and protected my siblings and me—by having everything they owned placed into their separate revocable living trusts. When our parents died, about 18 months apart, after my sibling who was the trustee paid their outstanding bills and any state inheritance taxes, our parents' assets were distributed exactly as stipulated in each of their identical trusts. The attorney's fees were minimal and everything transpired smoothly. My dad was a farmer and a wise businessman. On his advice, many years ago, my siblings and I similarly have protected our children by putting our assets into revocable living trusts.

The recommendations that follow are no substitute for the advice of a good lawyer. But friends and professionals alike have shared certain suggestions with me repeatedly, and I have experienced their value in my own family. I share them here to inspire you to begin the process of advance planning sooner rather than later so that you can enjoy life and not have to worry about these practical matters.

If, like my parents, you have a revocable living trust, at your death the trustee can distribute the assets in the trust without going through probate. If, instead, you own your assets in your sole name, on your death those assets will be subject to probate and oversight by the probate court. Because probate is a public process, the names of your beneficiaries, their addresses, any claims of your creditors, and a list of your probate assets are public record available to be reviewed at the local probate office. By contrast, *revocable living trusts are private*. There are other benefits, and some drawbacks, to transferring your assets to a revocable living trust and bypassing the probate process: One positive for creating such a trust is that a trust has a trustee who can distribute money or property, as directed for your care if you become incapacitated. And, after your death, the trustee can distribute funds to meet the needs of minor children, young adult children too immature to receive a lump sum estate payment, or adult disabled children who will require lifelong help with finances.

If you retain your assets in your name rather than transferring them to a revocable living trust, there are a number of ways that your assets will pass upon your death. Any jointly held property will pass to the joint owner at the moment of your death. Any assets with a beneficiary designation will pass to the named beneficiaries upon presentation of a death certificate to the holder of such asset. Beneficiaries of real property can be designated during your lifetime, reserving your ability to use the property but ensuring that it will become the property of the named beneficiary upon your death.

Finally, any asset in your name alone without beneficiary designation will be subject to probate, a process that generally takes between six and nine months. During that time the value of those assets are reported in an inventory, and an accounting is filed showing expenses, income, and sales during this period. The accounting also shows that the assets are distributed to those named in the will in the proportions designated. This could include a distribution to a trust for a minor or someone else who is unable to handle financial decision making. The beneficiaries of your estate get notice and can request copies of all of these filings.

The advantage of a revocable living trust is that at your death your assets can be distributed according to your wishes without the intervention of the probate court and without your information becoming public record. The advantage of having a will and your assets going through probate is that you (and your beneficiaries) have the assurance that your assets will be distributed according to your wishes, according to a mandated timetable, and that all information concerning assets and payments made are available for review. If assets are held in a revocable living trust, it would be more complicated to obtain relief from an uncooperative or slow to act trustee.

Your revocable living trust can be updated or changed by returning to an attorney who specializes in trusts. Even if you choose to use a revocable living trust, you still should have a will for any assets that inadvertently are omitted from the trust. Such a will would simply assign all such assets to the trustee of the revocable living trust. While a will can be contested in the probate court, a trust is rarely contested because it is legally quite hard to do. *In the absence of either a revocable living trust or a properly executed last will and testament, your assets will be distributed based on state law, and you will have no say in who receives them.*

The Documents You Need and Where to Keep Them

You will need—in your name—a revocable living trust or a last will and testament or both, an advance medical directive, a medical power of attorney, and durable power of attorney. (1) *The original copies of your trust and your will should be kept with your attorney and filed with the probate court for safe keeping.* (2) *Copies of each document need to be kept in a safe place in your home known to a trusted family member or friend, and also kept with the designated trustee of your trust and your durable power of attorney (this may be the same individual).* (3) It is a good idea to have duplicates on file in your financial advisor's office. (4) The individual designated to make medical decisions for you if you are incapacitated should have a copy of your medical power of attorney and advance medical directive and know where the original copy is available. A duplicate copy of your medical power of attorney and advance medical directive can be given to your physician prior to planned surgery or hospitalization. *Be sure to provide to those who need it the contact information of your lawyer and financial advisor. You should also keep an updated list of all of your passwords and account numbers in a secure place, accessible to your trustee in an emergency.*

If you decide to establish a revocable living trust, it is essential that you get retitled—in the name of your revocable living trust—each and all of your bank and investment accounts, and possibly also your home. Your retirement accounts (IRAs) cannot be transferred out of your name. Many advisors suggest that you get your insurance policies retitled so that the trust is listed as the beneficiary. Since relationships change principally due to death, divorce, and remarriage, *you need to review and, if necessary, update the beneficiary designations on your insurance policies, pension, and IRA accounts—so that, in the event of your incapacitation or death, your ex-spouse or deceased relative does not inherit these funds instead of your children or current spouse!* In the words of my own financial advisor, "No matter how sophisticated your plan, unless you title everything correctly, you can put the whole thing in a ditch!"

Beneficiary designations on insurance policies, IRAs, retirement assets, and certain others have legal precedence over the terms of a revocable living trust or will, and it is critical to keep them current. Designating a date once a year to review your documents can help accomplish this goal. If you have not transferred your assets to a revocable living trust and you do not have a will, then your assets will be distributed based on state law. This could be especially bad if an unintended heir is too young, a drug addict, or for some other reason might squander a great deal of money if it was inherited all at once. Instead, a trustee can distribute assets according to the trust in ways that protect each of the heirs. If the life insurance policy designates the revocable living trust or a trust established under your last will and testament as the beneficiary, the trustee can similarly protect each heir. *If you have been meaning to see an attorney about estate planning, this is a reminder to act.*

In my own experience with my parents, I was at times overwhelmed by all the details involved in the legal documents they needed—and blessedly had. The same is true now, as I put my own affairs in order to ease my daughters' tasks some day in the future. It isn't easy. It isn't fun. It's hard to discuss with my daughters because it makes them sad to think about my getting old if it's going to mean that I have impairments. And it's not something that my parents—or I—did on our own. We sought out professionals, triple-checked their credentials and reputations, and took their expert advice. (See appendix C for the needed contact information for other resources and practical guidance.)

IMPORTANT LEGAL DOCUMENTS

In addition to possibly needing a (1) *revocable living trust* (described earlier), you will need the legal documents described below to protect yourself and your loved ones:

(2) *An advance medical directive, also known as a living will/health care directive* specifies your medical preferences in the event of incapacitation due to illness or hospitalization: it states whether (a) you want your doctors to do absolutely everything to try to keep you alive (regardless of your condition), (b) you want nothing done other than to be kept comfortable, or (c) that you want nothing done other than artificially administered nutrition and hydration if necessary as well to be kept comfortable. The choice you make is applicable if your death is imminent from a terminal illness, you are in a persistent vegetative state, or you are in an end stage condition of a terminal illness.

(3) *A medical power of attorney* is the family member or family members, friend, physician, or group of designated persons to whom you legally give the authority to make the decisions regarding your advance medical directive *or* other medical decisions that are not life and death matters but are decisions needed in the event of your incapacitation.

(4) *A durable power of attorney* can be one person or more than one person, each designated for different decisions or transactions. A durable power of attorney can take several forms: *general* allows your representative to handle your financial and property-related affairs, *limited* gives the person decision-making authority over limited decisions that are spelled out, *durable* gives authority to your representative(s) to make decisions while you're still capable to make your own *or* after you become incapacitated or both.

(5) *A last will and testament* states how your property, possessions, assets, and debts are to be distributed when you die. This is usually necessary even if you also have a revocable living trust. Your will may be very simple or quite comprehensive, depending on whether you have a revocable living trust.

For information on choosing attorneys and advisors, see appendix C: Legal and Financial Resource Guide.

Long-Term Care Insurance

The cost of my father's nursing care was more than $100,000—in just the last 18 months of his life! Thankfully, my parents were frugal people, farmers who had lived through the Great Depression, so my siblings and I had our parents' savings to cover his care. Most people do not have the necessary $8,000 to $9,000 a month—the average cost of nursing care in a decently nice nursing facility—should a spouse or another loved one need such care. Most of us have to plan ahead in order not to place such a financial burden on our families.

At the age of 59, I personally decided to protect my daughters by purchasing long-term care insurance (LTC), a policy with an annual premium of $2,100, which just recently was raised to $2,600. (Premiums nationwide have been adjusted upward by all of the five or six major companies that still offer LTC policies because so many Americans are living longer, keeping their LTC policies, and using them.) I learned too late that had I bought a LTC policy at 50, my premiums would have been about half what I have paid up to now. My policy will pay a daily benefit of $314 for three years, should it be needed. This benefit can go toward in-home care, assisted living in the event of cognitive impairments or two of six functional impairments in daily living, or for a nursing home. Should I be blessed, as my parents were, to live into old old age (beyond 85), that is just about the time my children will start worrying about sending *their* children to college. While I look to my daughters for overseeing my care, I don't want to make their lives difficult financially.

A 47-year-old friend of mine has a husband who is 61 and is the son of parents who both lived long lives while needing nursing care for Alzheimer's disease. The couple is wisely looking into getting a long-term care policy for him. I am told by an insurance representative that he will probably pay about $2,200 per year for his policy—and likely not have increases in his premium due to the fact that insurance companies will have already reconfigured the cost, life expectancy, and claims factors that caused my premiums to rise.

My two closest friends since college—who are married to each other—decided *not* to purchase long-term care insurance because they have been able to save over the years, have pension income, and have each other to care for one another. Each individual and each couple must decide whether to get LTC insurance based on their own projected financial and health circumstances, and in consultation with their certified financial planner. (See appendix C in the back of his book.)

To study various long-term care insurance policies, be sure to identify several well-established insurance companies that have been in business many decades or longer, then Google their Comdex ratings (which will tell you how financially solid and user friendly each company is). You will want a company that writes long-term care polices and has a Comdex rating of 90 or more on a 100-point scoring system. Your certified financial planner can advise you far better than I can on the many factors to consider.

BRUCE: AFFIRMING LIFE, PLANNING AHEAD

He grew up in a Mennonite family, and attended an Amish Vacation Bible School. His mother was a full-time homemaker, and his dad was a state trooper with the Iowa Highway Patrol. One of Bruce's relatives started a Mennonite church out in the country, near where he was born—Eicher Emmanuel Mennonite Church—and both of his parents are buried in the cemetery there.

"When I was 5," Bruce recalls, "We went to a relative's funeral at a Lutheran church, and it was the first time I heard someone play the organ. I decided right then *that* was what *I* wanted to do." At the age of 7, he began taking piano lessons. At 12, he started organ lessons, paying for them with his paper route. He studied with musicians in the region who were the principal organists for their organizations. After a guest recitalist from Philadelphia came to the college he was attending in Iowa, he was invited to Philadelphia to audition, won a full scholarship to Curtis Institute of Music, and studied at one of the best schools for mastering the organ.

"I always knew I wanted to be involved in church choirs. Most of my life, I've had three jobs, two of them full time." At 84, Bruce recently retired after 55 years as the organist and director of music at one of the largest Methodist churches in Maryland and also retired after 28 years of full-time teaching at the prestigious Peabody Conservatory of the Johns Hopkins University.

Bruce has been blessed by the many opportunities to follow his vocational dreams. As a gay man, he has also been grateful for the love and support he has enjoyed from his colleagues and friends. For 53 years and counting, he continues to serve as the organist for a large conservative Jewish congregation. "I love the [two-hour] service," Bruce says, a Christian who more than once has considered converting to Judaism. "I love the thoughtful, warm people. The rabbis are gracious, and I have a great relationship with the Cantor. [The late] Rabbi

Loeb and I traveled together in Israel. He was a brilliant man, ahead of his time, a community leader who early on issued a warning about AIDS. His sermons were pastoral and generous in accepting gays. The people at the synagogue act like *Christians* are supposed to act! They are genuine friends who invite us into their homes and to share holidays. Members of the congregation don't hesitate to show their affection and appreciation. The rabbi after the service gave me a kiss on the cheek and said, 'Thank you, Bruce.' And the female rabbi walked by and pushed a cookie in my mouth while I was playing the service."

He particularly loves choral music. "That's when I feel closest to God. The chords, the harmony, and the words elevate my thoughts, my being. The sound of the organ just transports me."

Planning for the future and sharing helpful information with loved ones can be more complicated for those in the LGBTQ community, and that has been true for Bruce. "My first marriage, to a woman, lasted more than two decades, and I have three kids," Bruce explains. "After our divorce in 1976, we remained friends, sharing family celebrations for 26 years." Their middle child died of AIDS in 1992. Their daughter is 54 and lives locally. Their surviving son will be 60 next Christmas, is a retired chef, and lives with his wife in Phoenix. "I've got two blood grandkids and three step-grandkids."

From the age of 5, Bruce recalls knowing that something was different about him, "but I didn't have a name for it. When I went to college, I heard about gays, but I fought my sexuality for a long time. At 45, I decided that God made me this way. I'm going to be the best gay person I can be."

Bruce's partner is 61 years old. They've been together for 14 years. In 2002, when Bruce informed his former wife that he and Jorge had gone to Vermont to have a civil union ceremony, "she chose to stop all contact," Bruce told me, clearly wishing his friendship with the mother of his children could have continued. "The children chose not to attend our civil union, but since that time, they've come around and are very cordial to Jorge. We share holiday celebrations."

On January 3, 2013, Bruce and Jorge were married in Maryland, three days after it became legal. The opportunity to marry has been a significant help for same-sex couples, as they are able to take advantage of many spousal benefits that come automatically with marriage, including gaining the equal protection of inheritance laws. As for the 23-year age difference between them, Bruce has two perspectives. On one hand, "I tend to see everyone I deal with as older than me, and I'm younger than they are. I try to be agile whether I feel like it or not."

On the other hand, Bruce continues, "We are so much in love. My greatest fear is that I will sometime die and leave him." He has dealt with that fear proactively by taking care of his own health and completing the necessary advance planning documents.

Bruce says that his spouse "pushes me to go to the gym with him, and yells if I eat the wrong things." He "doesn't always pay attention" to his spouse's admonitions about eating healthier foods, but for the past 15 years Bruce does go to the gym five days a week. "It's a warm-water workout," he explains, "20 minutes of walking sideways, backward, and forward, plus some exercises that imitate running." Seventy years of practicing, performing, and playing the organ have taken a physical toll: because of "holding my back and neck erect in an unnatural way, I've had two back surgeries and kept a chiropractor in new cars and new homes." He has also had double bypass surgery and has a defibrillator. Regardless, most people would look at Bruce today and think of him as possibly in his middle 70s, not 10 years older.

The sea change that has come with the US Supreme Court's marriage equality ruling and society's changing attitudes toward gay and lesbian people, Bruce explains, has made it easier for him to protect his partner, given the likelihood that Bruce will die first. They jointly own their home, finally have spousal hospital visitation rights, and share spouse survival rights to their financial resources.

"I worked three jobs and saved money," Bruce says, "and whatever happens, I'll be okay." He has established the legal documents needed to protect himself and his loved ones: a living revocable trust, durable power of attorney, medical power of attorney, and an advance medical directive. Bruce's daughter, son, and spouse share the medical power of attorney; his best friend for 40 years is his executor; his son-in-law, a financial advisor by profession, is his second executor, and his lawyer is the third. "I have a loving daughter, son, and partner," Bruce says. Quoting the words from a favorite hymn, he adds, "Be not dismayed, whate'er betide, God will take care of you."

THE GIFT TO OUR LOVED ONES OF LIVING AN ACTIVE LIFE

Becoming a hermit is one of the most harmful things we can do to our brain as we get older, according to an April 8, 2011, study published online in the *Journal of the International Neuropsychological Society*. Following 1,138 adults with an average age of 80 for five years, the study found that "the most socially active seniors had just one-quarter the amount of cognitive decline as those who were the least social." Getting together with friends, going to religious services, volunteering, and engaging in regular cardio exercise—in summary, having an active social life plus getting our heart rates up by walking at a pace that is brisk but still slow enough to carry on a conversation—these are two of the most effective ways to try to "help stave off memory problems."[24]

In his television program produced for PBS, *Younger Next Year: The New Science of Aging*, Dr. Henry Lodge emphasizes *emotion* and *motion*. "If a man has had a heart attack, he has four times the risk of dying if he comes home [from the hospital] to an empty house, and half that risk if coming home to a dog" as his companion. "As mammals," Lodge says, "we work in packs, we're wired to work together." Attachment to others is "deeply rooted in our brains" for reasons of survival, and "emotion plays just as big a role as exercise." By getting off of our sofas and walking for 40 minutes, three times a week, we can reduce our risk of heart disease, diabetes, strokes, and dementia from other causes: "Fit people," he says, "have 40 percent less risk of Alzheimer's than unfit people."[25]

Remember, however, that many are unluckier than others with the genes they have inherited, toxins or head injuries or socioeconomic hardships or stressful life circumstances to which they've been exposed—all risk factors for dementia. For all of these reasons, it would be wrong to blame people, as if the responsibility for their brain health is entirely a matter of lifestyle. *It isn't.* Still, to whatever extent there is a "fountain of youth," regular exercise and strong, supportive relationships are the main reasons why many people look much younger than their actual years. Widely respected University of Michigan researcher Toni Antonucci calls physical activity "the right to move," and a "powerful, low-cost solution with positive benefits to cognitive, emotional, and physical health."[26]

When I lost my brother to cancer at the age of 77, it was a shock because our mother and father lived much longer lives and because Vaughn always took such good care of himself. For literally *decades* he exercised regularly, was health minded in his eating habits and overall lifestyle, and maintained strong family and friendship connections. What helped me bear the sorrow that my brother wasn't able to live a longer life was the clear realization that Vaughn lived a fuller life than many people who have lived into their 90s or beyond. This gift of comfort is something that each of us can leave to our surviving spouse, children, grandchildren, siblings, and friends. We can strive to be good people who count our blessings, make the most of our talents, and contribute to the betterment of others' lives. Most especially, we can leave a legacy of love to our family members. *We can live the best life within reach—regardless of the length of it.*

A MEANINGFUL LIFE

Whether illness, physical disability, dementia, or a premature death befalls us, what will most comfort our loved ones while we are alive and beyond—and aid them in moving forward after we're gone—is the knowledge that we did not live our lives accumulating regret.

When giving keynotes and other presentations, I often recommend a powerful little book full of wisdom entitled, *The Top Five Regrets of the Dying*, by Bronnie Ware. She is an Australian who gave palliative care to dying patients, in the last 3 to 12 weeks of their lives. The five most common regrets Ware heard spoken, again and again, were "(1) I wish I'd had the courage to live a life true to myself, not the life others expected of me. (2) I wish I didn't work so hard. (3) I wish I'd had the courage to express my feelings. (4) I wish I'd stayed in touch with my friends, and (5) I wish that I had let myself be happier."[27]

To me, the overarching message of Ware's dying patients is this: *happiness is a choice.* Allowing ourselves to be happy means making one decision after another: we can choose integrity; we can choose to value people over our work lives, while taking time to smell the roses; we can choose bravely to express our love and concern for others; and we can choose stay in close contact with our friends. By taking responsibility for finding or creating a meaningful life for ourselves, instead of blaming God, fate, life's hardships, or other people for our unhappiness, we can live and die without regret.

Finding meaning in life through connections with other people but also "a framework of values, a philosophy of life," writes Abraham Maslow, is something the human needs "in about the same sense as [he or she] needs sunlight, calcium, and love."[28] Meaning may also be found in "more mundane daily functions . . . habitual activities [and] everyday experiences of pleasure," add psychologists Samantha Heintzelman and Laura King.[29] Activities as simple as having one's morning coffee or evening dish of ice cream, listening to music, or watching sunrises, sunsets, the falling leaves of October, cloud formations, falling rain or snow, butterflies, birds and squirrels, or a favorite TV show—all of these simple pleasures can enrich our lives, as well.

Relevant here is an anonymous quote, framed and displayed in my office during the early years of my career, when I did counseling as a college chaplain: *"Let yourself get so attached to life that it can't give you up."* Choosing a full and happy life means deeply investing ourselves in relationships, with people, worthy causes, meaningful activities, or productive work, while appreciating nature's beauty and its creatures and living with thankful hearts. If we choose a way of life filled with gratitude and acts of kindness, the people we love don't have to be so sad at our funerals!

"Religion and spirituality may be an underappreciated resource," as well, and "a form of meaningful social participation" that has even been shown to reduce the risk of suicide among American women.[30] "Religious convictions and practices can help people foster a sense of hope, even in the midst of major crises or adversities," writes Aaron Kheriaty, a professor of psychiatry at the University of California Irvine. "Religious faith can help people find a sense of meaning and purpose even in suffering."[31]

From the age of 20, when I first read his book *Man's Search for Meaning*, Viktor Frankl has profoundly influenced my life. He was a 37-year-old physician, a psychiatrist, when his papers came through and he could have fled Austria to the United States in 1942, but he hadn't wanted to leave his elderly parents. All members of his family were deported to different Nazi concentration camps, and he endured three years in four different death camps. On being liberated, Frankl learned that his pregnant wife, both parents, his brother, his best friend, and many of his friends who were also doctors had perished in the Holocaust. All alone and battling despair, he rewrote the manuscript the Nazis had forcibly taken from him and destroyed, then added his own and others' experiences of imprisonment, degradation, torture, and death. This book would be published in 24 languages, and is still read widely 70 years later. A college student, learning for the first time about the unspeakable evil, savage cruelty, and horrors of the Holocaust, I knew that whatever lessons Dr. Frankl had to share about the meaning of life were lessons so authentic that I had to learn them.

"Each person must choose the way in which he bears his burden," Frankl wrote. "Forces beyond your control can take away everything you possess except one thing, your freedom to choose how you will respond to the situation." Frankl lived another 52 years!

He married his second wife, headed up the neurology department at a hospital in Vienna for 25 years, lectured many times on every continent, published many works, visited the United States 63 times, held professorships at Harvard, Stanford, and the University of Pittsburgh, and always returned to live in his beloved Austria. He was 92 when he died, having lectured just two years earlier to an international gathering of professionals representing medicine, psychology, philosophy, and religion.[32]

There are three main paths for arriving at a sense of meaning in one's life, according to Viktor Frankl: we find a life worth living by (1) creating a work or doing a deed, (2) loving someone, and most importantly (3) rising above a hopeless situation, refusing to be a victim of a fate we are helpless to change and by *changing ourselves* to turn a personal tragedy into a triumph.[33]

THE MANY REWARDS OF CAREGIVING

So many women and men have shared with me the growing they have done and the deep sense of purpose they have found in taking care of their loved ones. Frankl was right: our lives are given meaning from the work and good deeds we do, the love we give, and the ways we grow stronger through hard, challenging times.

Because of your caring, kindness, and the sacrifices *you* have made, you are giving your loved one and yourself more happy times together. The memories of these good times will stay with you when the difficult, painful times begin to fade in your mind and grow increasingly distant.

You can be proud of yourself for the many ways you've learned to cope with difficult situations. You can respect yourself for each and every way you have tried to find the best life within reach in such stressful, often sad times. As you've made sacrifices to help your loved one, you've been *helping yourself* to become a better person.

In the words of former First Lady Rosalynn Carter, "There are only four kinds of people in the world: those who have been caregivers; those who are currently caregivers; those who will be caregivers; and those who will need caregivers."[34] Still one last reward of caregiving, yet to be realized, is that you may be modeling patience and kindness—problem-solving skills and loving care—to those who someday will take care of you!

Epilogue

A LETTER TO MY DAUGHTERS

Dearest Daughters,

However long I live, in whatever ways I remain healthy and strong or become ill or grow frail, there are some things I hope you will always remember. More than anything, I want you to remember that being your mom is the best thing that could ever have happened to me. Loving and being loved by you, delighting in each of you as babies and little girls, and being so proud of you as young women—nothing will ever top that for giving meaning to my life and warmth to my heart.

I hope to be able to live well into my 90s with the sharp mind and physical mobility that Betty, my bridge-playing friend, has and with the resilience to overcome physical disabilities and the love of lifelong learning seen in Aunt Dorris—both of them born 20 years ahead of me. But if for some reason that level of mental acuity, physical strength, quality and length of life isn't the life I'm able or given to enjoy, I want you to remember that I have *already* lived a full and happy life. Like each of you, I was loved unconditionally by my mother and grandmother. Like you, I had some amazing teachers, mentors, learning experiences, and travel opportunities. Like you, as a child and as an adult, I have had pets that I loved, countless activities that I've enjoyed, and an untold number of reasons to live with a thankful heart.

With these blessings come responsibilities. Like you, I got to grow up in a wonderfully diverse and beautiful country with the strongest democracy in the world, learned from my parents a strong work ethic, earned a good education, was never hungry or homeless, and had access to needed health care. Like me, you know that we've had these and other blessings that many Americans still don't have, and that billions of people around the world don't have even their most basic needs met. I know that each of you lives thankfully, and I hope you will always look for ways to care for and help people less fortunate.

Through some very difficult losses over the years, I've been able to heal and grow stronger because caring friends, colleagues, ministers, mentors, and therapists helped me and inspired me to help others. My life also is greatly enriched from having married once, fallen in love twice again, and being blessed with long-lasting, loving relationships with wonderful friends. Since the age of 19, when I began to support myself through college, I have wanted my life to count for good in others' lives. Thankfully, I have had more than 50 years of rewarding, meaningful work—so satisfying and fulfilling that I still don't want to retire. What a tremendous and ongoing blessing are all of these years of teaching, writing, counseling, occasionally leading religious services (even some funerals), and giving lectures, workshops, and media presentations all over this country. I'm grateful for every single opportunity that came my way and every person who offered support and encouragement. But the absolutely most rewarding and precious gift in my life will always remain sharing *your* lives and being your mama.

If it should happen some day that I become physically impaired or gradually develop Alzheimer's disease like my mother / your grandma—who never stopped being sweet, appreciative, loving, and spiritually strong—I hope to be like her! From reading this book, however, you will know that people whose dementia is more advanced than your grandma's illness are *not* in control of their emotions and behavior. Whatever happens, I trust you to make the best decisions on my behalf that you can, should that responsibility fall to you. If these decisions are hard or cannot restore what is lost through illness or disability, please don't feel guilty. Just keep in mind this quote from the Dalai Lama: *"Whenever possible, be kind. It is always possible."* And don't forget to be kind to yourselves!

I've done my best to put in place the documents and provide the resources needed for you to help me when I'm old (an advance medical directive, all the legal documents I've advised others to have, plus long-term care insurance, and a financial plan for retirement). If you read and reread chapter 12, you will have much information and sensitivity to the quality of life issues in old age that I hope you will keep in mind for my sake. It is my fervent hope that your *own* children and husbands will care for *you* in disability or old age with similar knowledge, sensitivities, and perspectives.

My heart will thank God until my dying day for the deeply fulfilling gift of being your mom and having *you* as my daughters! Please take good care of yourselves and of each other.

With much love,

Mom

APPENDIX A

Helpful Books and Videos

FOR FURTHER READING

Here are some of the best books I came across while writing my own book—
resources with helpful knowledge, practical guidance, and valuable insights for
caregivers of an older adult.

On Caring for Your Loved One

Being Mortal: Medicine and What Matters in the End, by Atul Gawande. New
York: Henry Holt, 2014.

Coping with Alzheimer's: A Caregiver's Emotional Survival Guide, by Rose
Oliver and Frances A. Bock. New York: Dodd, Mead, 1987.

Coping with Your Difficult Older Parent, by Grace Lebow and Barbara Kane.
New York: HarperCollins, 1999.

Creating Moments of Joy for the Person with Alzheimer's or Dementia, by Jolene
Brackey. West Lafayette, IN: Perdue University Press, 2016.

How to Care for Your Aging Parents, by Virginia Morris. New York: Workman,
2014.

I'm Still Here: A New Philosophy of Alzheimer's Care, by John Zeisel. New York:
Avery, 2010.

Learning to Speak Alzheimer's, by Joanne Koenig Coste. New York: Houghton
Mifflin Harcourt, 2003.

A Loving Approach to Dementia Care, by Laura Wayman. 2nd ed. Baltimore:
Johns Hopkins University Press, 2017.

*Loving Someone Who Has Dementia: How to Find Hope While Coping with Stress
and Grief*, by Pauline Boss. San Francisco: Jossey-Bass, 2011.

The 36-Hour Day, by Nancy L. Mace and Peter V. Rabins. 6th ed. Baltimore:
Johns Hopkins University Press, 2017.

Treating Dementia in Context: A Step-by-Step Guide, by Susan M. McCurry and
Claudia Drossel. Washington, DC: American Psychological Association
Press, 2011.

When a Family Member Has Dementia, by Susan M. McCurry. New York:
Praeger Press, 2006.

On Caring for Yourself as You Age

Meditations for Women Who Do Too Much, by Anne Wilson Schaef. San Francisco: HarperCollins, 1990.

The Top Five Regrets of the Dying, by Bronnie Ware. Australia: Hay House,
2012.

Use Your Brain to Change Your Age, by Daniel G. Amen. New York: Crown
Archetype Press, 2012.

VIDEOS

I also found a number of helpful videos, some of them available online, some
as DVDs. Sometimes, after a hard day, you may find viewing a video easier than
picking up another book. And you may find that viewing a video gives you a
perspective reading can't. See what works for you.

Aging Backwards, with Miranda Esmonde-White. *Classical Stretch by Essentrics*,
PBS. DVD. www.essentrics.com/classicalstretch.html.

*Brain Fit: 50 Ways to Grow Your Brain with Daniel Amen, MD, and Tana Amen,
RN*, Mindworks Production, pledge program for PBS, November 25,
2016–December 31, 2018. DVD available through your local public television station.

Caregiver Support: Survival Tips for Caring for Elderly Parents, with Dr. Christiane Northrup. drnorthrup.com.

Change Your Brain, Change Your Life with Dr. Daniel Amen. PBS. High Five
Entertainment, 2015. DVD. info@epstv.com.

Glorious Women Never Age, with Christiane Northrup, 2015. Five-minute
preview and DVD. wgbh.org.

The Happiness Advantage, with Shawn Achor. Twin Cities Public Television /
Tremendous Entertainment, 2012. DVD.

Younger Next Year: The New Science of Aging, with Henry S. Lodge. Advise &
Consent / PBS Distribution, 2011. DVD.

Finally, there are even more choices you can find in the online listing from the
Alzheimer's Association Recommended List of Videos: https://www.alz.org
/library/downloads/resources_library_recommended_videos2015.pdf.

Additional Resources

There are as many types of caregivers as there are types of people—and there are many different types of resources and organizations available. I've gathered together all that I could find, in hopes of helping you find some sources of help that meet your needs and the needs of the loved one you are caring for. (Descriptions in quotations marks are taken directly from the websites.)

INFORMATION ON AGING

Administration on Aging (Administration for Community Living)

"The OAA promotes the well-being of older individuals by providing services and programs designed to help them live independently in their homes and communities. The Act also empowers the federal government to distribute funds to the states for supportive services for individuals over the age of 60."

(202) 401-4634
aclinfo@acl.hhs.gov
www.aoa.gov

American Geriatrics Society

"The American Geriatrics Society (AGS) is a not-for-profit organization of nearly 6,000 health professionals devoted to improving the health, independence and quality of life of all older people. The Society provides leadership to healthcare professionals, policy makers and the public by implementing and advocating for programs in patient care, research, professional and public education, and public policy."

(212) 308-1414
info.amger@americangeriatrics.org
www.americangeriatrics.org

American Society on Aging

The American Society on Aging seeks "to support the commitment and enhance the knowledge and skills of those who seek to improve the quality of life of older adults and their families."

(800) 537-9728

www.asaging.org

The Gerontological Society of America

GSA's mission "is to advance the study of aging and disseminate information among scientists, decision makers, and the general public."

(202) 842-1275

www.geron.org

Leading Age (formerly American Association of Homes and Services for the Aging)

"Leading Age's Consumer Hub offers information and support to help people make the most of the aging experience. This includes a directory of not-for-profit organizations committed to meeting people's needs and preferences as they age."

(202) 783-2242

info@leadingage.org

http://www.leadingage.org

National Asian Pacific Center on Aging

NAPCA helps Asian elders with "many unique challenges, including cultural and language barriers and access to services and employment opportunities."

Chinese: (800) 582-4218

Korean: (800) 582-4259

Vietnamese: (800) 582-4336

English: (800) 336-2722

www.napca.org

National Association for Hispanic Elderly

The National Association for Hispanic Elderly (Asociación Nacional Pro Personas Mayores) work "includes employment programs, services for the elderly, economic development projects which include low-income housing and neighborhood development programs, research and data collection, training and technical assistance, development of model projects, and award winning media productions."

(626) 564-1988

www.anppm.org

National Association of Area Agencies on Aging

N4A is a "membership association representing America's national network of 622 Area Agencies on Aging (AAAs) and providing a voice in the nation's capital for the 256 Title VI Native American aging programs."

www.n4a.org

National Caucus and Center on Black Aging

"NCBA is one of the country's oldest organizations dedicated to aging issues and the only national organization devoted to minority and low-income aging."

(202) 637-8400

www.ncba-aged.org

National Council on Aging

NCOA is "a respected national leader and trusted partner to help people aged 60+ meet the challenges of aging. We partner with nonprofit organizations, government, and business to provide innovative community programs and services, online help, and advocacy."

(571) 527-3900

www.ncoa.org

National Hispanic Council on Aging

"NHCOA has been a strong voice dedicated to promoting, educating, and advocating for research, policy, and practice in the areas of economic security, health, and housing for more than 30 years." It also "is the leading national organization working to improve the lives of Hispanic older adults, their families and their caregivers."

(202) 347-9733

www.nhcoa.org

National Indian Council on Aging

"The mission of NICOA is to advocate for improved comprehensive health, social services, and economic well-being for American Indian and Alaska Native Elders."

(505) 292-2001
www.nicoa.org

National Resource Center on LGBT Aging

"The National Resource Center on LGBT Aging provides training, technical assistance and educational resources to aging providers, LGBT organizations and LGBT older adults."

(212) 741-2247
info@lgbtagingcenter.org
www.lgbtagingcenter.org

Services & Advocacy for Gay, Lesbian, Bisexual, and Transgender Elders (SAGE)

"SAGE is a national organization that offers supportive services and consumer resources for LGBT older adults and their caregivers, advocates for public policy changes that address the needs of LGBT older people, and provides training for aging providers and LGBT organizations, largely through its National Resource Center on LGBT Aging."

(212) 741-2247
info@sageusa.org
www.sageusa.org

RESOURCES FOR PEOPLE WITH DISABILITIES

Disability.gov

Disability.gov is a government website that "connects people with disabilities, their families and caregivers to helpful resources on topics such as how to apply for disability benefits, find a job, get health care or pay for accessible housing."

www.disability.gov

Paralyzed Veterans of America

"Paralyzed Veterans of America, a congressionally chartered veterans service organization founded in 1946, has developed a unique expertise on a wide variety of issues involving the special needs of our members—veterans of the armed forces who have experienced spinal cord injury or disease."

Caregiver Support: (855) 260-3274
Healthcare Helpline: (800) 232-1782
info@pva.org
www.pva.org

MEDICAL DISEASE RESEARCH, SUPPORT, AND SERVICES (NON-ALZHEIMER'S)

American Academy of Family Physicians

"The mission of the AAFP is to improve the health of patients, families, and communities by serving the needs of members with professionalism and creativity."

(800) 274-2237
aafp@aafp.org
www.aafp.org

American Diabetes Association

An organization with the mission "to prevent and cure diabetes and to improve the lives of all people affected by diabetes."

1-800-DIABETES / (800) 342-2383
www.diabetes.org

Arthritis Foundation

"We lead the fight for the arthritis community through life-changing information and resources, access to optimal care, advancements in science and community connections."

(844) 571-HELP / (844) 571-4357
www.arthritis.org

The Brain Injury Association of America

"BIAA's mission is to advance awareness, research, treatment, and education and to improve the quality of life for *all* people affected by brain injury. We are dedicated to increasing access to quality health care and raising awareness and understanding of brain injury."

National Brain Injury Information Center: (800) 444-6443
www.biausa.org

BrightFocus

"At BrightFocus, we support research to end Alzheimer's disease, macular degeneration, and glaucoma."

(800) 437-2423
info@brightfocus.org
www.brightfocus.org

National Alliance on Mental Illness

"NAMI, the National Alliance on Mental Illness, is the nation's largest grassroots mental health organization dedicated to building better lives for the millions of Americans affected by mental illness."

NAMI Helpline: (800) 950-6264
http://www.nami.org

DEMENTIA & ALZHEIMER'S RESEARCH, SUPPORT, AND TREATMENT

Alzforum

"Founded in 1996, Alzforum is a news website and information resource dedicated to helping researchers accelerate discovery and advance development of diagnostics and treatments for Alzheimer's disease and related disorders."

contact@alzforum.org
www.alzforum.org

Alzheimer's Association

The Alzheimer's Association "advances research to end Alzheimer's and dementia while enhancing care for those living with the disease."

24/7 helpline: (800) 272-3900
info@alz.org
www.alz.org

Alzheimer's Association Resource Finder

"Get easy access to a comprehensive listing of Alzheimer's and dementia resources, community programs and services."

24/7 helpline: (800) 272-3900
www.communityresourcefinder.org

Alzheimer's Foundation of America

The mission of the Alzheimer's Foundation of America (AFA) is "to provide optimal care and services to individuals confronting dementia, and to their caregivers and families through our member organizations dedicated to improving quality of life."

(866) 232-8484
www.alzfdn.org

Alzheimers.gov

Alzheimers.gov is "the government's free information resource about Alzheimer's disease and related dementias. Here you can find links to authoritative, up-to-date information from agencies and organizations with expertise in these areas."

(877) 696-6775
www.alzheimers.gov

American Psychological Association

"APA is the leading scientific and professional organization representing psychology in the United States. Our mission is to advance the creation, communication and application of psychological knowledge to benefit society and improve people's lives."

(800) 374-2721
(202) 336-5500
www.apa.org

Fisher Center for Alzheimer's Research Foundation

"The Fisher Center is one of the largest and most modern scientific facilities in the world dedicated to solving the puzzle of Alzheimer's disease."

800-ALZINFO / (800) 259-4636
info@alzinfo.org
www.alzinfo.org

Johns Hopkins Memory and Alzheimer's Treatment Center

"The Memory and Alzheimer's Treatment Center is a collaborative partnership between the departments of psychiatry, neurology, and geriatric medicine that offers patients comprehensive evaluation and innovative treatment to patients with a range of conditions that affect cognition and memory, including Alzheimer's disease and other dementias, traumatic brain injury, and brain vascular disease."

Clinic Information: (410) 550-6337
Research Clinical Trials: (410) 550-9054
Community Outreach: (410) 550-2281

An especially valuable resource also at Johns Hopkins Medicine is available at http://www.hopkinsmedicine.org/health/healthy_aging/caregiver_resources /facing-dementia-in-the-family.

Lewy Body Dementia Association

"The Lewy Body Dementia Association (LBDA) is a 501(c)(3) nonprofit organization dedicated to raising awareness of the Lewy body dementias (LBD), supporting people with LBD, their families and caregivers and promoting scientific advances."

(800) 539-9767
www.lbda.org

National Institute of Neurological Disorders and Stroke

As part of the National Institutes of Health, the mission of NINDS is to seek fundamental knowledge about the brain and nervous system and to use that knowledge to reduce the burden of neurological disease.

(800) 352-9424
www.ninds.nih.gov

National Rehabilitation Information Center

"The National Rehabilitation Information Center (NARIC) is the library of the National Institute on Disability, Independent Living, and Rehabilitation Research (NIDILRR). We collect, catalog, and disseminate the articles, reports, curricula, guides, and other publications and products of the research projects funded by NIDILRR. NIDILRR funds more than 250 projects each year that conduct research on a wide range of issues including technology, health and function, independent living, and capacity building."

(800) 346-2742
naricinfo@heitechservices.com
www.naric.com

University of California, San Francisco, Frontotemporal Dementia

"UCSF's Memory and Aging Center (MAC) actively conducts research and clinical trials to improve the diagnosis and treatment of FTD—and even search for a cure."

www.memory.ucsf.edu/ftd

CAREGIVER TOOLS AND SUPPORT

Aging Networks

Aging Networks describe themselves as "geriatric care managers and psychotherapists" with clients "who feel a strong sense of responsibility to parents who can no longer function independently. They are determined to keep their parents safe and as high-functioning as possible."

www.agingnets.com

ALZwell Caregiver Support

ALZwell Caregiver Support "helps people who are caring for individuals with Alzheimer's Disease and related Dementias to improve quality of life by providing practical information on the diagnosis, treatment, care and management of the disease."

(631) 224-7262
prisminnovations@gmail.com
www.alzwell.com

Caregiver Action Network

"CAN serves a broad spectrum of family caregivers ranging from the parents of children with special needs, to the families and friends of wounded soldiers; from a young couple dealing with a diagnosis of MS, to adult children caring for parents with Alzheimer's disease."

(202) 454-3970
info@caregiveraction.org
www.caregiveraction.org

CareZone

"CareZone makes it simpler to take care of yourself and your family. Keep everything organized and easily coordinate with the people that matter to you."

www.carezone.com

Caring Bridge

"Caring Bridge helps you create a free personal website to quickly share updates about your own or someone else's health journey."

www.caringbridge.org

Caring.com

Caring.com provides "personal, one-on-one guidance with a Family Advisor, thousands of original articles, helpful tools, a comprehensive local Senior Care Directory, and the collective wisdom of an involved community. Caring.com's carefully researched and expert-reviewed content includes advice from a team of more than 50 trusted leaders in geriatric medicine, law, finance, housing, and other key areas of healthcare and eldercare."

(650) 312-7100
www.caring.com

Family Caregiver Alliance

"The services, education programs, and resources FCA provides are designed with caregivers' needs in mind and offer support, tailored information, and tools to manage the complex demands of caregiving."

(800) 445-8106
www.caregiver.org

Lotsa Helping Hands

"With the Help Calendar, you can post requests for support—things like meals for the family, rides to medical appointments, or just stopping by to visit."

www.lotsahelpinghands.com

National Alliance for Caregiving

"National Alliance for Caregiving is a non-profit coalition of national organizations focused on improving the lives of family caregivers."

(301) 718-8444
info@caregiving.org
www.caregiving.org

National Caregiver's Library

"Find hundreds of articles, forms, checklists and links to topic-specific external resources."

www.caregiverslibrary.org

Rosalynn Carter Institute for Caregiving

The Rosalynn Carter Institute for Caregiving is "an advocacy, education, research, and service unit of Georgia Southwestern State University."

(229) 928-1234
www.rosalynncarter.org

Tyze

"Tyze is an online tool that brings people together around someone receiving care."

info@tyze.com
www.tyze.com

VA Caregiver Support

This site is part of the US Department of Veterans Affairs and offers information and support for veterans and their caregivers.

Veterans Crisis Line: (800) 273-8255
VA's Caregiver Support Line: (855) 260-3274
www.caregiver.va.gov

Well Spouse Association

This organization "offer[s] peer to peer support and educate[s] health care professionals and the general public about the special challenges and unique issues 'well' spouses face every day."

(800) 838-0879
www.wellspouse.org

ELDERCARE SERVICES

AAA Senior Driving

Part of the American Automobile Association website "dedicated to keeping seniors driving for as long and as safely possible."

www.seniordriving.aaa.com

AARP

"AARP is a nonprofit, nonpartisan, social welfare organization with a membership of nearly 38 million that helps people turn their goals and dreams into real possibilities, strengthens communities and fights for the issues that matter most to families—such as health care, employment and income security, and protection from financial abuse."

(888) OUR-AARP / (888) 687-2277
member@aarp.org
www.aarp.org
AARP en Español: http://www.aarp.org/espanol/
AARP Caregiving: http://www.aarp.org/home-family/caregiving/
AARP Long-Term Care Calculator: http://www.aarp.org/relationships
    /caregiving-resource-center/LTCC/?intcmp=FTR-LINKS-CRGVNG-LTCC
    -EWHERE
AARP Black Community: http://www.aarp.org/home-family/voices/black
    -community/
AARP Asian American and Pacific Islander Community: http://www.aarp
    .org/home-family/voices/asian-community/?cmp=RDRCT-AE
    -ASNCOMMUNITY-022216

Aging Life Care Association

"Aging Life Care™, also known as geriatric care management, is a holistic, client-centered approach to caring for older adults or others facing ongoing health challenges. Working with families, the expertise of Aging Life Care Professionals provides the answers at a time of uncertainty."

(520) 881-8008
http://www.aginglifecare.org

Aging with Dignity

A private nonprofit organization that is a "trusted resource for people who want to plan for care in advance of a health crisis. Our Five Wishes document is the most widely used advance directive or living will in America."

(888) 5WISHES / (800) 594-7437
fivewishes@agingwithdignity.org
www.agingwithdignity.org

The Alzheimer's Store

"The Alzheimer's Store is proud to offer a wide range of Alzheimer's products to ease patient's suffering and help them live in a safer home environment with a sense of security."

(800) 752-3238
contact@alzstore.com
www.alzstore.com

Argentum

"Argentum is the leading national trade association serving companies that own, operate, and support professionally managed senior living communities in the United States. Through a network of state partners, Argentum represents over 7,000 communities that provide independent living, assisted living, and memory care services for seniors."

(703) 894-1805
info@argentum.com
http://www.argentum.org/alfa/default.asp

BenefitsCheckUp

"BenefitsCheckUp is a free service of the National Council on Aging (NCOA), a nonprofit service and advocacy organization in Arlington, VA. Benefits-CheckUp asks a series of questions to help identify benefits that could save you money and cover the costs of everyday expenses."

(571) 527-3900
www.benefitscheckup.org

Eldercare Locator

Eldercare Locator is "a public service of the U.S. Administration on Aging connecting you to services for older adults and their families."

(800) 677-1116
www.eldercare.gov

Experience Works

"Experience Works is a national nonprofit organization whose mission is to improve the lives of older people through training, community service, and employment."

www.experienceworks.org

Medicaid

"Medicaid provides health coverage to millions of Americans, including eligible low-income adults, children, pregnant women, elderly adults and people with disabilities. Medicaid is administered by states, according to federal requirements. The program is funded jointly by states and the federal government."

(877) 267-2323
www.medicaid.gov

Medicare

Find health and drug plans, hospitals, doctors, service providers, suppliers of medical supplies and equipment, and information about Medicare plans.

(800) 633-4227
www.medicare.gov

National Adult Day Services Association

NADSA "members include adult day center providers, associations of providers, corporations, educators, students, retired workers and others interested in working to build better lives for adults in adult day programs every day."

(877) 745-1440
info@NADSA.org
www.nadsa.org

National Adult Protective Services Association

The mission of NAPSA "is to strengthen the capacity of [Adult Protective Services] at the national, state, and local levels, to effectively and efficiently recognize, report, and respond to the needs of elders and adults with disabilities who are the victims of abuse, neglect, or exploitation, and to prevent such abuse whenever possible."

(217) 523-4431
www.napsa-now.org

National Meals on Wheels Association of America

"Meals on Wheels America is the oldest and largest national organization supporting the more than 5,000 community-based senior nutrition programs across the country that are dedicated to addressing senior hunger and isolation. This network exists in virtually every community in America and, along with more than two million volunteers, delivers the nutritious meals, friendly visits and safety checks that enable America's seniors to live nourished lives with independence and dignity."

(888) 998-6325
www.mowaa.org

National PACE Association

"The National PACE Association (NPA) advances the efforts of Programs of All-Inclusive Care for the Elderly (PACE®). PACE programs coordinate and provide all needed preventive, primary, acute and long-term care services so older individuals can continue living in the community."

(703) 535-1565
info@npaonline.org
www.pace4you.org

National State Health Insurance Assistance Program (SHIP) Resource Center

"The State Health Insurance Assistance Program, or SHIP, is a national program that offers one-on-one counseling and assistance to people with Medicare and their families."

www.shiptalk.org

New Lifestyles

New Lifestyles provides "comprehensive, quality information on senior residences and care options."

(800) 869-9549
newlife@newlifestyles.com
www.newlifestyles.com

OWL

"OWL uses education, research and advocacy to be the voice of women over 40."

(202) 450-8986
info@owl-national.org
www.owl-national.org

A Place for Mom

"A Place for Mom connects moms, dads, seniors and families like yours to the right elder care so you can have peace of mind and focus on your loved ones."

(206) 285-4666
www.aplaceformom.com

Senior Corps

"The Senior Corps offers volunteer opportunities and services to people who are 55 years of age and older. The program consists of three main parts. The RSVP program, the Foster Grandparent program and the Senior Companion program."

www.seniorcorps.org

SeniorJobBank

"The SeniorJobBank, very simply, is a meeting place for over-50 job seekers and the employers seeking their services."

www.seniorjobbank.org

SeniorNet

"SeniorNet's mission is to provide older adults (the underserved) education for and access to computer technologies to enhance their lives and enable them to share their knowledge and wisdom."

(239) 275-2202
members@hq.seniornet.org
www.seniornet.org

Supplemental Nutrition Assistance Program (SNAP)

"SNAP offers nutrition assistance to millions of eligible, low-income individuals and families and provides economic benefits to communities."

www.fns.usda.gov/snap

thirdAGE

"ThirdAGE provides thoughtfully curated health and lifestyle content, offering a full-range of interactive up-to-the-moment information—including video, slideshows, health condition centers, articles about cutting-edge research and more—all medically reviewed and approved by our team of thirdAGE physicians." Information is targeted at women 45+ years of age.

www.thirdage.com

This Caring Home

Find information about making your home safer and easier to live in for people with dementia.

support@thiscaringhome.org
www.thiscaringhome.org

LIFESTYLE AND HOBBIES

Alzheimer's Poetry Project

"The mission of the [Alzheimer's Poetry Project] is to improve the quality of life of people living with Alzheimer's disease and related dementia by facilitating creative expression through poetry."

garyglaznerpoet@gmail.com
www.alzpoetry.com

National Senior Games Association

The NSGA is a "non-profit corporation dedicated to promoting healthy and active lifestyles for athletes age 50 and over."

(225) 706-5101
nsga@nsga.com
www.nsga.com

Road Scholar

For eligible caregivers, Road Scholar can help "you offset the costs of arranging substitute care while you attend a Road Scholar learning adventure through our Caregiver Grants."

(800) 454-5768
contact@roadscholar.org
www.roadscholar.org/about/financial-assistance/caregiver-grants/

LONG-TERM AND HOSPICE CARE

The American Elder Care Research Organization

"The website is designed to help families and caregivers locate information about long-term care resources for their loved ones, and to find the public and private programs available to assist in covering the cost of such care."

(641) 715-3900
www.payingforseniorcare.com

CaringInfo

"CaringInfo, a program of the National Hospice and Palliative Care Organization, provides free resources to help people make decisions about end-of-life care and services before a crisis."

(800) 658-8898
caringinfo@nhpco.org
www.caringinfo.org

Hospice Foundation of America

HFA provides "programs for professional development, public education and information; funding research, producing publications, and by providing information on issues related to hospice and end-of-life care."

(800) 854-3402
https://hospicefoundation.org

National Association for Home Care and Hospice

"The National Association for Home Care & Hospice (NAHC) is the largest and most respected professional association representing the interests of chronically ill, disabled, and dying Americans of all ages and the caregivers who provide them with in-home health and hospice services."

(202) 547-7424
www.nahc.org

National Consumer Voice for Quality Long-Term Care

"The Consumer Voice is the leading national voice representing consumers in issues related to long-term care, helping to ensure that consumers are empowered to advocate for themselves. We are a primary source of information and tools for consumers, families, caregivers, advocates and ombudsmen to help ensure quality care for the individual."

(202) 332-2275
info@theconsumervoice.org
www.theconsumervoice.org

National Hospice and Palliative Care

This organization "is committed to improving end of life care and expanding access to hospice care with the goal of profoundly enhancing quality of life for people dying in America and their loved ones."

(703) 837-1500
nhpco_info@nhpco.org
www.nhpco.org

Psychologists in Long-Term Care

"Psychologists in Long-Term Care is a network of psychologists and other professionals dedicated to the enhancement of mental health and quality of life for those involved in long-term care through practice, research and advocacy."

www.pltcweb.org

Legal and Financial Resource Guide

CHOOSING A LAWYER WITH EXPERTISE IN TRUSTS, WILLS, AND ESTATE PLANNING

Before you choose a lawyer, there are several questions you need to ask: (1) What experience do you have with writing revocable living trusts, working for whom, how many years? (2) What are your qualifications? (3) What will I pay you to write my living revocable trust? My advance medical directive, also known as a living will / health care directive? Medical power of attorney? Durable power of attorney? Last will and testament? (4) Have you ever been publicly disciplined for any unlawful or unethical actions during your professional career?*

Be sure you get—and understand—answers to each question. Having a lawyer who can explain all the complications in ways you can understand is key.

CHOOSING AND USING A CERTIFIED FINANCIAL PLANNER

A good certified financial planner (CFP) is not just someone who will talk with you about your present needs and future goals for saving and investing money; he or she will work with you to be sure that "the big picture" of your family's life is secure both financially and legally. Your CFP should annually review with you (and keep updated copies on file) of your living revocable trust, will and amendments to the will, durable power of attorney, health care power of attorney, insurance policies (including for long-term care), tax returns (past two years), and current income, savings, and benefits statements.

My trusted CFP does even more. In addition to all of the above, he has a list of my emergency and key contacts (family, friends, physician, attorney), lists of my assets, any loans or debt, my saving needs for retirement, my daughters' education and weddings, and my future grandchildren.

---

* The author has adapted this material from CFP, "Other Financial Planning Resources," http://www.letsmakeaplan.org/other-resources/selecting-an-advisor.

Whether you've gotten the name of a potential CFP from a trusted friend or colleague (the best way to start) or from an online search to find a CFP in your region, you can verify that person's credentials through the website of the Certified Financial Planner Board of Standards. Online, in person, or by phone, you'll need the answers to these questions: (1) What experience do you have, working for whom, for how many years? (2) What are your qualifications, and do you have the certified financial planner (CFP) certification? (3) What financial planning services do you offer, and what is your approach to financial planning? (4) What types of clients do you typically work with? (5) Will you be the only financial planner working with me? (6) What will I pay for your financial planning services, and how much do you typically charge? (7) Have you ever been publically disciplined for any unlawful or unethical actions during your professional career?*

If your CFP is investing money for you, you'll also need to write up an investment policy statement that outlines the general rules you want your manager to follow. It is a statement of your goals and objectives and describes the strategies you want your manager to employ: How do you want your assets allocated? How much risk are you comfortable with at this time in your life? How much of your money do you need to have readily available (liquidity requirements, assets that can be bought and sold without losing money)? Do you have any *social constraints* (opposition to investments related to alcohol, tobacco, firearms, or companies that engage in animal testing) or social *preferences* (such as investments in renewable energy sources)?†

---

* Ibid.

† CFP, "What a Certified Financial Planner Professional Can Do for You," http://www.letsmakeaplan.org/why-choose-a-cfp-professional.

Notes

Chapter 1. The Challenge

1. R. Acierno, M. A. Hernandez, A. B. Amstadter, H. S. Resnick, K. Steve, W. Muzzy, et al., "Prevalence and Correlates of Emotional, Physical, Sexual, and Financial Abuse and Potential Neglect in the United States: The National Elder Mistreatment Study," *American Journal of Public Health* 100 (2010): 292–97; L. B. Schiamberg, G. G. Barboza, J. Oehmke, Z. Zhang, R. J. Griffore, R. P. Weatherhill, et al., "Elder Abuse in Nursing Homes: An Ecological Perspective," *Journal of Elder Abuse and Neglect* 23 (2011): 190–211.

2. Viktor Frankl, *Man's Search for Meaning* (New York: Washington Square Press, 1963).

3. JoAnn T. Tschanz, Kathleen Piercy, Chris D. Corcoran, Elizabeth Fauth, Maria C. Norton, Peter V. Rabins, Brian T. Tschanz, M. Scott Deberard, Christine Snyder, Courtney Smith, Lester Lee, and Constantine G. Lyketsos, "Caregiver Coping Strategies Predict Cognitive and Functional Decline in Dementia: The Cache County Dementia Progression Study," *American Journal of Geriatric Psychiatry* 21 (January 2013): 1.

4. E. K. Kababgambe, S. E. Judd, V. J. Howard, et al., "Inflammation Biomarkers and Risk of All-Cause-Mortality in the Reasons for Geographic and Racial Differences in Stroke (REGARDS) Cohort," *American Journal of Epidemiology* 174, no. 3 (2011): 284–92; N. Christakis and P. Allison, "Mortality after the Hospitalization of a Spouse," *New England Journal of Medicine* 354, no. 7 (2006): 719–30; Marcia C. Ory, Richard R. Hoffman III, Jennifer L. Yee, Sharon Tennstedt, and Richard Schulz, "Prevalence and Impact of Caregiving: A Detailed Comparison between Dementia and Non-dementia Caregivers," *Gerontologist* 39, no. 2 (1999): 177–85; Arline T. Geronimus, Margaret Hicken, Danya Keene, and John Bound, "'Weathering' and Age Patterns of Allostatic Load Scores among Black and Whites in the United States," *American Journal of Public Health* 96, no. 5 (May 2006): 826–33.

5. Elizabeth Fauth, Kyle Hess, Maria Northon, Chris Corcoran, Peter Rabins, Constantine Lyketsos, and JoAnn Tschanz, "Caregivers' Relationship Closeness with the Person with Dementia Predicts Both Positive and Negative Outcomes for Caregivers' Physical Health and Psychological Well-Being," *Aging and Mental Health* 16, no. 6 (August 2012): 699–711.

6. David L. Roth, William E. Haley, Martha Hovater, Martinique Perkins, Virginia G. Wadley, and Suzanne Judd, "Family Caregiving and All-Cause Mortality: Findings from a Population-Based Propensity-Matched Analysis," *American Journal of Epidemiology* 178, no. 10 (2013): 1571–78; Michael J. Poulin, Stephanie L. Brown, Amanda J. Dillard, and Dylan M. Smith, "Giving to Others and the Association between Stress and Mortality," *American Journal of Public Health* 103, no. 9 (2013):1649–55; Michael J. Poulin, Stephanie L. Brown, Peter A. Ubel, Dylan M. Smith, Aleksandra Jankovic, and Kenneth M. Langa, "Does a Helping Hand Mean a Heavy Heart? Helping Behavior and Well Being among Spouse Caregivers," *Psychology and Aging* 25, no. 1 (March 2010): 108–17.

7. Sun Woo Kang and Nadine F. Marks, "Filial Caregiving Is Associated with Greater Neuroendocrine Dysfunction: Evidence from the 2005 National Survey of Midlife in the U.S.," *SAGE Open Medicine*, January 30, 2014, journals.sagepub.com /doi/full/10.1177/2050312113520152; R. Mahoney, C. Regan, C. Ktona, and G. Livingston, "Anxiety and Depression in Family Caregivers of People with Alzheimer Disease: The LASER-AD Study," *American Journal of Geriatric Psychiatry* 13, no. 9 (September 2005): 795–801; Helga Ask, Ellen Melbye Langballe, Jostein Holmen, Geir Selbaek, Ingvild Saltvedt, and Kristian Tambs, "Mental Health and Well Being in Spouses of Persons with Dementia: The Nord-Trondelag Health Study," *BMC Public Health* 14 (2014): 413; N. R. Nielsen, T. S. Kristensen, P. Schnohr, M. Gronback, "Perceived Stress and Cause Specific Mortality among Men and Women: Results of a Prospective Cohort Study," *American Journal of Epidemiology* 168, no. 5 (2008): 481–91; Elissa Epel, "How Chronic Stress Is Harming Our DNA," *Monitor on Psychology*, October 2014, 28–31.

8. Roth et al., "Family Caregiving and All-Cause Mortality."

9. Poulin et al., "Giving to Others and the Association between Stress and Mortality," 1652.

10. Cretien van Campen, Alice H. de Boer, and Jurjen Ledema, "Are Informal Caregivers Less Happy Than Noncaregivers? Happiness and the Intensity of Caregiving in Combination with Paid and Voluntary Work," *Scandinavian Journal of Caring Sciences* 27, no. 1 (2012), 44–50, doi:10.1111/j.1471–6712, emphasis mine.

11. Laura E. Berk, *Development Through the Lifespan*, 6th ed. (New York: Pearson, 2014), 550.

12. Robert M. Sapolsky, *Why Zebras Don't Get Ulcers—a Guide to Stress, Stress-Related Disorders and Coping*, 3rd ed. (New York: W. H. Freeman, 2004); Linda L. Barrett, *Caregivers: Life Changes and Coping Strategies* (Washington, DC: AARP Research, 2013).

13. Berk, *Development*, 549–50.

14. Ory et al., "Prevalence and Impact of Caregiving," 177–85.

15. Berk, *Development*, 549–50.

16. Ory et al., "Prevalence and Impact of Caregiving," 179.

17. S. L. Brown, D. M. Smith, et al., "Caregiving Behavior Is Associated with Decreased Mortality Risk," *Psychological Science* 20 (2009): 488–94; also cited by M. J. Poulin et al., "Does a Helping Hand Mean a Heavy Heart?"

18. Poulin et al., "Does a Helping Hand Mean a Heavy Heart?," 111.

19. Gail M. Williamson, David R. Shaffer, and Richard Schulz, "Activity Restriction and Prior Relationship History as Contributors to Mental Health Outcomes among Middle-Aged and Older Spousal Caregivers," *Health Psychology* 17, no. 2 (1998): 152–62.

20. Ibid.

21. Ibid.

22. Gail M. Williamson and Richard Schulz, "Relationship Orientation, Quality of Prior Relationship, and Distress among Caregivers of Alzheimer's Patients," *Psychology and Aging* 3, no. 4 (1990): 502–9.

23. Sherman A. James, Nora L. Keenan, David S. Strogatz, Steven R. Browning, and Joanne M. Garrett, "Socioeconomic Status, John Henryism, and Blood Pressure in Black Adults: The Pitt County Study," *American Journal of Epidemiology* 135, no. 1 (1992): 59–67.

24. M. A. Subramanyam, S. A. James, A. V. Diez-Roux, et al., "Socioeconomic

Status, John Henryism and Blood Pressure among African Americans in the Jackson Heart Study," *Social Science Medicine* 93 (September 2013): 139–46.

25. "John Henryism Key to Understanding Coping, Health," *Duke Medicine News and Communications* 2006, https://corporate.dukehealth.org/news-listing/%E2%80 %98john-henryism%E2%80%99-key-understanding-coping-health?h=nl.

26. Peggye Dilworth-Anderson, Ishan Canty Williams, and Brent E. Gibson, "Issues of Race, Ethnicity, and Culture in Caregiving Research: A 20-Year Review (1980–2000)," *Gerontologist* 42, no. 2 (2002): 237–72.

27. Ibid.

28. Jung-Hyun Kim and Bob G. Knight, "Effects of Caregiver Status, Coping Styles, and Social Support on the Physical Health of Korean American Caregivers," *Gerontologist* 48, no. 3 (2008): 287–99.

29. K. A. Roberto and S. E. Jarrott, "Family Caregivers of Older Adults: A Life Span Perspective," *Family Relations* 57 (2008): 100–11. Also Berk, *Development*, 551.

30. Berk, *Development*, 567–68.

31. Professor William Haley is quoted from Paula Spencer Scott's article, "The Unexpected Joys of Caregiving," in the *AARP Bulletin*, November 2014, www.aarp.org /home-family/caregiving/info-2014/caregiving-happiness-confidence-compassion .html.

Chapter 2. On Both Sides, Vulnerability and Loss

1. *Oxford English Dictionary* (1993).

2. Laura E. Berk, *Development Through the Lifespan*, 6th ed. (New York: Pearson, 2014).

3. *AARP Bulletin*, September 2014.

4. Anna Gorman, "Helping Families Cope with a Loved One's Fading Memory," *Washington Post*, March 5, 2014.

5. Mark was one of my mentors, too, hiring me for my first job out of seminary to be his associate chaplain at a large university—when women simply had no chance of being hired for such roles and no churches of my denomination in that state would have accepted a woman minister. I will always be grateful for Mark's paramount influence in my life, including his encouragement of my subsequent writing and teaching career. Although Mark and Laura and I have lived geographically apart for more than 40 years, we've stayed close. I love, deeply respect, cherish, and think of them as my brother and sister.

6. Cecilia Brennecke, quoted in "When an Aging Mom Becomes the Child," Health and Science, *Washington Post*, April 9, 2013.

7. John Schneider, "Helping Grieving Families Help Themselves" (speech given at Kellogg Center, Michigan State University, East Lansing, Michigan, October 1, 1984).

8. Brennecke, quoted in "When an Aging Mom Becomes the Child."

9. Google Books' earliest credit: someone in an Alcoholics Anonymous meeting in 1993. Nelson Mandela is said to have spoken similar words many years earlier.

10. Shawn Achor, *The Happiness Advantage* (Twin Cities Public Television / Tremendous Entertainment, 2012), DVD jacket cover content description.

11. Ibid.

12. Ibid.

Chapter 3. Is This Normal Aging or Dementia?

1. American Psychiatric Association, *Diagnostic and Statistical Manual of Mental Disorders*, 5th ed. (*DSM-5*) (Arlington, VA: American Psychiatric Association, 2013), 608. In contrast to major neurocognitive disorder, the *DSM-5* further explains that "estimates of the prevalence of mild cognitive impairment (. . . mild NCD) among older individuals are fairly variable, ranging from 2% to 10% at age 65 and 5% to 25% by age 85 . . . Very late in life, cognitive symptoms may not cause concern or may go unnoticed. In late life, mild NCD must also be distinguished from the more modest deficits associated with 'normal aging,' although a substantial fraction of what has been ascribed to normal aging likely represents prodromal phases of various NCDs" (608–9).

2. Dr. Wattenbarger managed human performance engineering organizations at Bell Labs and AT&T laboratories. In 2015, I interviewed him for his expertise regarding complex reasoning tasks.

3. Laura E. Berk, *Development Through the Lifespan*, 6th ed. (New York: Pearson, 2014), 568.

4. L. L. Heston, *Mending Minds: A Guide to the New Psychiatry of Depression, Anxiety, and Other Serious Mental Disorders* (New York: W. H. Freeman, 1992). Excerpts quoted in Ronald J. Comer, *Fundamentals of Abnormal Psychology*, 8th ed. (New York: Worth, 2016), 501.

5. Heston, *Mending Minds*, 87–90; Comer, *Fundamentals of Abnormal Psychology*, 501.

6. Nancy L. Mace and Peter V. Rabins, *The 36-Hour Day*, 6th ed. (Baltimore: Johns Hopkins University Press, 2017), 24, 7.

7. Ibid., 25.

8. Fredrick Kunkle, "Alzheimer's Signs and Some False Alarms," *Baltimore Sun*, April 16, 2015.

9. Fredrick Kunkle, "Early Alzheimer's in Parent Exacts Heavy Toll on Young Adult Children," *Washington Post*, January 28, 2015.

10. Christiane Northrup, *Glorious Women Never Age*, KPBS TV, May 30, 2015.

11. Becca R. Levy, Alan B. Zonderman, Martin B. Slade, and Luigi Ferrucci, "Memory Shaped by Age Stereotypes over Time," *Journal of Gerontology: Psychological Sciences* 67, no. 4 (2012): 432–36.

12. Chris Kelly, "McCartney Goes from Fab Four to Spry 74," *Washington Post*, August 11, 2016.

13. Bruce Fretts, "Sidney Poitier—His Life of Turmoil and Triumph," *Closer* 4, no. 45 (November 7, 2016), 21–24.

14. Northrup, *Glorious Women Never Age*.

Chapter 4. Aging as Successfully as Possible—Both You and Your Loved One

1. Laura E. Berk, *Development Through the Lifespan*, 6th ed. (New York: Pearson, 2014), 518.

2. Ibid., 596.

3. Stephen F. Barnes, *Third Age—the Golden Years of Adulthood* (San Diego, CA: San Diego State University Interwork Institute, 2011).

4. Paul Wink and Jacquelyn Boone James, "Conclusion: Is the Third Age the Crown of Life?," *Annual Review of Gerontology and Geriatrics* 26 (2006): 305.

5. Berk, *Development*, 596.

6. Jacqui Smith and Paul B. Baltes, "Trends and Profiles of Psychological Functioning in Very Old Age," in *The Berlin Aging Study—Aging from 70 to 100*, ed. Paul B. Baltes and Karl Ulrich (New York: Cambridge University Press, 1999), 197–226.

7. Paul B. Baltes and Jacqui Smith, "New Frontiers in the Future of Aging: From Successful Aging of the Young Old to the Dilemmas of the Fourth Age," *Gerontology* 49 (2003): 123–35; Mike Yassa, "Advances in Preventing Cognitive Decline: Getting Old, Thinking Young; Institute for Brain Potential" (workshop presented in Baltimore, Maryland, 2013), and others say that Alzheimer's affects "one in two after age 85 [not age 90]."

8. Baltes and Smith, "New Frontiers," 123–35, emphasis mine.

9. George E. Vaillant and Kenneth Mukamal, "Successful Aging," *American Journal of Psychiatry* 158, no. 6 (2001): 839. *Merriam-Webster* defines "oxymoron" as "a combination of contradictory or incongruous words (as cruel kindness)."

10. Vaillant and Mukamal, "Successful Aging," 839.

11. K. I. Erickson, C. A. Raji, O. L. Lopez, J. T. Becker, et al., "Physical Activity Predicts Gray Matter Volume in Late Adulthood: The Cardiovascular Health Study," *Neurology* 75, no. 16 (2010): 1415–22.

12. Pew Research Center Social and Demographic Trends, "Growing Old in America: Expectations vs. Reality," June 29, 2009, www.pewsocialtrends.org/2009/06/29/growing-old-in-america-expectations-vs-reality.

13. Corey L. Keys and Gerben J. Westerhof, "Chronological and Subjective Age Differences in Flourishing Mental Health and Major Depressive Episode," *Aging and Mental Health* 16, no. 1 (2012): 67–74.

14. Ibid.

15. Kirsten M. Wilkins, "Sexuality and Aging: The New Normal," presentation given at Sheppard Pratt Hospital in Baltimore, May 6, 2015. Wilkins is an MD and associate professor of psychiatry at Yale University School of Medicine. See also L. J. Waite, E. O. Laumann, A. Das, and L. P. Schumm, "Sexuality: Measures of Partnerships, Practices, Attitudes, and Problems in the National Social Life, Health and Aging Study," *Journal of Gerontology* 64B (2009): i.56–i.66.

16. Pew Research Center, "Growing Old in America," 5.

17. Ibid.

18. Becca Levy, M. D. Slade, T. E. Murphy, and T. M. Gill, "Association between Positive Age Stereotypes and Recovery from Disability in Older Persons," *Journal of the American Medical Association* 308, no. 19 (November 21, 2012): 1972–73.

19. Judith Graham, "Older People Become What They Think," *New York Times*, December 19, 2012.

20. Ros Altmann, "Who Are You Calling Old? Let's Ditch Ageist Stereotypes," *Guardian*, February 4, 2015, www.the guardian.com/society/2015/feb/04/old-ditch-ageist-stereotypes. According to Nancy R. Peppard, PhD, in "An Essay on Myths and Stereotypes," written for the Oregon Department of Human Services in June 2012, "the term 'ageism' was coined by [geriatrician] Robert Butler, M.D., in 1968 . . . Butler felt ageism is a form of bigotry that is a very serious national problem."

21. Dana Kotter-Grühn and Thomas M. Hess, "The Impact of Age Stereotypes on Self-Perceptions of Aging Across the Adult Lifespan," *Gerontology Series B Psychological Sciences and Social Sciences* 67 (2012): 563–71.

22. Miranda Esmonde-White, *Aging Backwards: Classical Stretch by Essentrics*, PBS, www.essentrics.com/classicalstretch.html.

23. Baltes and Smith, "New Frontiers," 311–37.

24. Ibid.

25. Ibid.

26. Dan Rodricks, "Almost 109, and Still Going Strong, Honey," *Baltimore Sun*, October 29, 2016.

27. Alice Park, Melissa August, Anne Berryman, Hanna Kite, Chris Lambie, Jeff Israely, and Francis X. Rocca, "How to Live to Be 100," *Time*, August 30, 2004, 40–47.

28. American Psychiatric Association, *Diagnostic and Statistical Manual of Mental Disorders*, 5th ed. (Arlington, VA: American Psychiatric Association, 2013), 631.

29. A. Ott, R. P. Stolk, F. van Harskamp, A. Hofman, and M. M. B. Breteler, "Diabetes Mellitus and the Risk of Dementia," *Neurology* 53 (1999): 1937–941.

30. K. I. Erickson, C. A. Raji, O. L. Lopez, J. T. Becker, et al., "Physical Activity Predicts Gray Matter Volume in Late Adulthood: The Cardiovascular Health Study," *Neurology* 75, no. 16 (2010): 1415–22.

31. Gretchen Reynolds, "A Little Exercise for the Mind," *New York Times*, August 18, 2015.

32. J. Verghese, B. Lipton, M. J. Katz, et al., "Leisure Activities and the Risk of Dementia in the Elderly," *New England Journal of Medicine* 348, no. 25 (June 19, 2001): 2508–16.

33. C. Thomas and C. I. Baker, "Teaching an Adult Brain New Tricks: A Critical Review of Evidence for Training-Dependent Structural Plasticity in Humans," *Neuroimage* 73 (June 2013): 225–36. Also Linda Searing, "Mentally Challenging Work May Protect Your Brain Late in Life," *Washington Post*, May 5, 2015; Linda Searing, "Jobs That Stimulate the Brain May Have a Later-in-Life Payoff," *Washington Post*, November 25, 2015; Jon Saraceno, "A Bridge to Brain Power: Playing Your Cards Right Can Help Keep You Sharp Long after Retirement," *AARP Bulletin*, March 2015, www.aarp.org/health/brain-health/info-2015/bridge-for-brain-health.html.

34. Daniel G. Amen, *Use Your Brain to Change Your Age* (New York: Crown Archetype Press, 2012), 60–61.

35. Laura E. Berk, *Development Through the Lifespan*, 6th ed. (New York: Pearson, 2014), 551, 587, 586, 623, 624. Also Jung-Hyun Kim and Bob G. Knight, "Effects of Caregiver Status, Coping Styles, and Social Support on the Physical Health of Korean American Caregivers," *Gerontologist* 48, no. 3 (2008): 287–99; Colleen Anne Richard and Alison Hamilton Brown, "Configurations of Informal Social Support among Older Lesbians," *Journal of Women and Aging* 18, no. 4 (2006): 49–65.

36. Nancy L. Mace and Peter V. Rabins, *The 36-Hour Day*, 6th ed. (Baltimore: Johns Hopkins University Press, 2017), 371, 372.

37. *Change Your Brain, Change Your Life with Dr. Daniel Amen*, PBS (High Five Entertainment, 2015), DVD, info@epstv.com, based on the book by Daniel G. Amen, *Change Your Brain, Change Your Life* (New York: Harmony Books, 1998; New York: Penguin Random House, 2015).

Chapter 6. Caregiver Stress—What Helps and What Usually Doesn't

1. Rosemary Blieszner and Karen Roberto, "Care Partner Responses to the Onset of Mild Cognitive Impairment," *Gerontologist* 20, no. 1 (2010): 11–22.

2. Ibid.

3. Ibid.

4. JoAnn T. Tschanz, Kathleen Piercy, Chris D. Corcoran, Elizabeth Fauth, Maria C. Norton, Peter V. Rabins, Brian T. Tschanz, M. Scott Deberard, Christine Snyder, Courtney Smith, Lester Lee, and Constantine G. Lyketsos, "Caregiver Coping Strategies Predict Cognitive and Functional Decline in Dementia: The Cache County Dementia Progression Study," *American Journal of Geriatric Psychiatry* 21, no. 1 (2013): 57–66; Christine M. Snyder, Elizabeth Fauth, Joseph Wanzek, Kathleen W. Piercy, Maria C. Norton, Chris Corcoran, Peter V. Rabins, Constantine G. Lyketsos, and JoAnn T. Tschanz, "Dementia Caregiver Coping Strategies and Their Relationship to Health and Well-Being: The Cache County Study," *Aging & Mental Health* 15, no. 5 (2014): 390–99.

5. Tschanz et al., "Caregiver Coping Strategies," 57–66.

6. Virginia Morris, *How to Care for Your Aging Parents* (New York: Workman, 2014), 39.

7. Ibid.

8. Angela Beasley Freeman, *100 Years of Women's Wisdom: Timeless Insights from Great Women of the 20th Century* (Nashville, TN: Walnut Grove Press, 1999), 65.

9. Ibid., 64.

10. Quran, *Al-Isra'* [The night journey], trans. Maulana Wahiduddin Khan, ed. Farida Khanam (New Delhi: Goodword Books, 2009), 210 verses 23–24.

11. Shraga Simmons, "ABCs of Honoring Parents," www.aish.com/f/hp/48964606 .html.

12. Ibid.

13. Laura E. Berk, *Development Through the Lifespan*, 6th ed. (New York: Pearson, 2014), 249.

14. Ibid., 551.

15. Tschanz et al., "Caregiver Coping Strategies," 57–66.

16. Susan M. McCurry, *When a Family Member Has Dementia* (New York: Praeger Press, 2006); Susan M. McCurry and Claudia Drossel, *Treating Dementia in Context: A Step-by-Step Guide* (Washington, DC: American Psychological Association Press, 2011).

17. Susan M. McCurry, "Treating Dementia in Context: Understanding the Big Picture in Dementia Care" (talk presented at OGEC Alzheimer's Disease Education Workshop, Oregon Geriatric Education Center, Portland, Oregon, April 3, 2014). Available on YouTube at https://youtube.com/watch?v=aCVUvFBjem0. The slides from this talk are available at ohsu.edu/xd/education/schools/school-of-nursing/about/centers /oregon-geriatric-education/upload/OGEC-2014_McCurry.pdf.

18. Ibid.

19. This quote from Dr. DePaulo and the one that follows were part of an early conversation at the Johns Hopkins University School of Medicine and Hospital, when I sought the chief of psychiatry's advice early in the writing of this book.

20. Susan Hannah Hadary and William Whiteford, producers, William Whiteford, director, *Grace: The Alzheimer's Documentary* (Baltimore, MD: Video Press), DVD, September 24, 2012.

21. Linda Teri, *Managing and Understanding Behavior Problems in Alzheimer's Disease and Related Disorders* (training program with videotapes and written manual) (Seattle: University of Washington, 1990).

22. McCurry, "Treating Dementia in Context: Understanding the Big Picture in Dementia Care."

23. McCurry, *When a Family Member Has Dementia*.

24. McCurry and Drossel, *Treating Dementia in Context*, 2011.

25. "Intensive Caregivers," *AARP Bulletin*, November 2015, 14.

26. Ibid.

27. Ibid.

28. Ibid.

29. Paula Spencer Scott, "Places That Lend a Hand," *AARP Bulletin*, November 2015, 16.

30. Dale A. Lund, Robert D. Hill, Michael S. Caserta, and Scott D. Wright, "Video Respite: An Innovative Resource for Family, Professional Caregivers, and Persons with Dementia," *Gerontologist* 35 (October 1995): 5; "Alzheimer's Respite Video—Mom Watching for the Very First Time," YouTube video, posted by Toni Wombaker, August 14, 2012, https://www.youtube.com/watch?v=nIbe00M3yzA.

31. "Random Acts of Kindness for Caregivers," *AARP Bulletin*, November 2015, 14.

32. Berk, *Development*, 587; Lund et al., "Video Respite," 5.

33. Linda J. Barrett, "Caregivers: Life Changes and Coping Strategies," *AARP Research* (2013), www.aarp.org/content/dam/aarp/research/surveys_statistics/general/2013/Caregivers-Life-Changes-and-Coping-Strategies-AARP-rsa-gen.pdf, 8–9.

34. Susan McCurry's PowerPoint presentation of April 24, 2013, slide number 52.

35. This is something of a paraphrase from the above-cited McCurry presentation, "Treating Dementia in Context." Slide number 51 reads, "No matter how slow you go, you are still lapping everybody on the couch." The second sentence is a paraphrase of McCurry's slide number 61.

36. Berk, *Development*, 587.

Chapter 7. Comforting Insights and Myth-Busting Knowledge

1. Shawn Achor, *The Happiness Advantage* (Twin Cities Public Television / Tremendous Entertainment, 2012), DVD.

2. John Zeisel, *I'm Still Here: A New Philosophy of Alzheimer's Care* (New York: Avery, 2010), 55–56.

3. Ibid., 56.

4. Ibid., 62.

5. Dr. Rodolfo "Rudy" Zea is a Maryland psychologist and humanist interested primarily in geriatrics and the aging process from a clinical standpoint. Dr. Zea shared his professional experiences and insights with me in a personal conversation in 2015, Towson, Maryland.

6. JoAnn T. Tschanz, Kathleen Piercy, Chris D. Corcoran, Elizabeth Fauth, Maria C. Norton, Peter V. Rabins, Brian T. Tschanz, M. Scott Deberard, Christine Snyder, Courtney Smith, Lester Lee, and Constantine G. Lyketsos, "Caregiver Coping Strategies Predict Cognitive and Functional Decline in Dementia: The Cache County Dementia Progression Study," *American Journal of Geriatric Psychiatry* 21, no. 1 (2013): 57–66.

7. Janice Lynch Schuster, "When the Mind Starts to Go," *Washington Post*, April 9, 2013.

8. Ibid. Schuster quotes Lisa Snyder, *Living Your Best with Early-Stage Alzheimer's* (North Branch, MN: Sunrise River Press: 2010).

9. Joe Breighner, *For the Love of Stray Cats* (Baltimore: FATA, 2000), 16.

Chapter 9. Truly Helpful Caregiving Tips

1. Susan Berger, "How to Talk to a Friend Who Has Alzheimer's," *Washington Post*, May 31, 2016.

2. Ibid. Berger is quoting Ruth Drew, director of family and information services at the Alzheimer's Association.

3. Ibid.

4. Joanne Koenig Coste, *Learning to Speak Alzheimer's* (New York: Houghton Mifflin Harcourt, 2003), 37.

5. Ibid.

6. Laura Wayman, *A Loving Approach to Dementia Care* (Baltimore: Johns Hopkins University Press, 2011), 51–54.

7. Ibid.

8. Nancy L. Mace and Peter V. Rabins, *The 36-Hour Day*, 6th ed. (Baltimore: Johns Hopkins University Press, 2017), 26, emphasis in original.

9. Atul Gawande, *Being Mortal: Medicine and What Matters in the End* (New York: Henry Holt, 2014), 105. Here Gawande quotes Keren Brown Wilson and describes her pioneering accomplishments.

10. Ibid., 105. These powerful words are Gawande's own.

11. Coste, *Learning to Speak Alzheimer's*, 92.

12. Ibid., 119.

13. Claudia Miranda-Castillo, Bob Woods, and Martin Orrell, "The Needs of People with Dementia Living at Home from User, Caregiver and Professional Perspectives: A Cross-Sectional Survey," *BMC Health Services Research* 13, no. 1 (2013): 1.

14. John Zeisel, *I'm Still Here: A New Philosophy of Alzheimer's Care* (New York: Avery, 2010), 140.

15. Mace and Rabins, *36-Hour Day*, 236, 240–241.

16. Rose Oliver and Frances A. Bock, *Coping with Alzheimer's: A Caregiver's Emotional Survival Guide* (New York: Dodd, Mead, 1987), 202–3.

17. Ibid., 47.

18. Ibid.

19. Ibid.

20. Susan M. McCurry and Claudia Drossel, *Treating Dementia in Context: A Step-by-Step Guide* (Washington, DC: American Psychological Association, 2011), 138.

21. Ibid.

22. Ibid., 141.

23. Ibid.

24. Ibid., 58.

25. Ibid.

26. Debbie Reslock, "The Cruelty of Calling Older Adults 'Sweetie' or 'Honey,'" *Huffington Post*, November 1, 2016.

27. Ibid.

28. McCurry and Drossel, *Treating Dementia in Context*, 58.

29. Anne Wilson Schaef, *Meditations for Women Who Do Too Much* (San Francisco: HarperCollins, 1990), September 14 meditation.

30. Ibid., November 13 meditation; Gawande, *Being Mortal*, 105.

31. Jolene Brackey, *Creating Moments of Joy for the Person with Alzheimer's or Dementia* (West Lafayette, IN: Perdue University Press, 2007), 114. Brackey's book is now out in a 2017 edition as *Creating Moments of Joy along the Alzheimer's Journey*.

32. JoAnn T. Tschanz, Kathleen Piercy, Chris D. Corcoran, Elizabeth Fauth, Maria C. Norton, Peter V. Rabins, Brian T. Tschanz, M. Scott Deberard, Christine Snyder, Courtney Smith, Lester Lee, Constantine G. Lyketsos, "Caregiver Coping Strategies Predict Cognitive and Functional Decline on Dementia: The Cache County Dementia Progression Study," *American Journal of Geriatric Psychiatry* 21, no. 1 (2013): 57–66.

33. Tschanz et al., "Caregiver Coping Strategies"—making the point about the need for caregiver and care recipient engagement in daytime activities and companionship, in order to reduce behavioral symptoms and caregiver burden—cites Peter V. Rabins, Nancy L. Mace, and M. J. Lucas, "The Impact of Dementia on the Family," *JAMA* 248 (1982): 333–35.

34. Schaef, *Meditations for Women Who Do Too Much*, November 13 meditation.

35. Tschanz et al., "Caregiver Coping Strategies," 62.

36. McCurry and Drossel, *Treating Dementia in Context*, 58.

37. Oliver and Bock, *Coping with Alzheimer's*, 174.

38. Jolene Brackey, *Creating Moments of Joy*, 114.

39. Pauline Boss, *Loving Someone Who Has Dementia: How to Find Hope While Coping with Stress and Grief* (San Francisco: Jossey-Bass, 2011), 165.

Chapter 10. When Your Loved One Dies—Relief, Grief, and Moving Forward

1. Grace Lebow and Barbara Kane, *Coping with Your Difficult Older Parent* (New York: HarperCollins, 1999), 191.

2. Ralph Keyes, *Chancing It* (Boston: Little, Brown, 1985), 154–55, 284.

Chapter 11. What Kind of an "Old Person" Will I / Will You Become?

1. Becca R. Levy, Martin D. Dale, and Thomas M. Gill, "Hearing Decline Predicted by Elders' Stereotypes," *Journal of Gerontology: Psychological Sciences* 61, no. 2 (2006): P82–P87. Also Becca R. Levy and Erica Leifheit-Limson, "The Stereotype-Matching Effect: Greater Influence on Functioning When Age Stereotypes Correspond to Outcomes," *Psychology and Aging* 24, no. 1 (2009): 230–33; Thomas M. Hess and Joey T. Hinson, "Age-Related Variation in the Influences of Aging Stereotypes on Memory in Adulthood," *Psychology and Aging* 21, no. 3 (September 2006): 621–25; Becca R. Levy, Martin D. Slade, Terrence E. Murphy, Thomas M. Gill, "Association between Positive Age Stereotypes and Recovery from Disability in Older Persons," *JAMA* 308, no. 19 (November 2012): 1972–73.

2. Laura E. Berk, *Development through the Life Span*, 6th ed. (New York: Pearson, 2014), 573.

3. Henry S. Lodge, *Younger Next Year: The New Science of Aging* (Advise & Consent / PBS Distribution, 2011), DVD.

4. Levy, Dale, and Gill, "Hearing Decline Predicted by Elders' Stereotypes," 82–87.

5. Berk, *Development*, 568.

6. "Older Adults with Hearing Loss Who Use Hearing Aids Perform Significantly Better on Cognitive Tests Than Those Who Do Not Use Hearing Aids," In Brief, *Monitor on Psychology* 47 (July/August 2016): 7, 16.

7. Yale University, "Negative Beliefs about Aging Predict Alzheimer's Disease in Study," *Science Daily*, December 7, 2015, www.sciencedaily.com/releases/2015/12/151207145906.htm. Also Becca R. Levy, Luigi Ferrucci, Alan B. Zonderman, Martin D. Slade, Juan Troncoso, and Susan M. Resnick, "A Culture-Brain Link: Negative Age Stereotypes Predict Alzheimer's Disease," *Psychology and Aging* 31, no. 1 (February 2016): 82–88.

8. Berk, *Development*, 574. Also Becca R. Levy, Martin D. Slade, Stanislav V. Kasl, and Suzanne R. Kunkel, "Longevity Increased by Positive Self-Perceptions of Aging," *Journal of Personality and Social Psychology* 83, no. 2 (2002): 261–70.

9. Margy Rochlin, "Leading Ladies," *AARP—the Magazine* 59, no. 4C (June/July 2016): 34–37.

10. Toni C. Antonucci and Hiroko Akiyama, "Stress and Coping in the Elderly," *Applied and Preventive Psychology* 2 (1993): 201–8.

11. Kahlil Gibran, *The Prophet* (New York: Knopf, 1961), 19.

12. Bruce Evan Blaine, *Understanding the Psychology of Diversity* (Los Angeles: Sage, 2013), 186. The two or three of the "forms of retirement" described here come from the work of Kenneth Shultz and Mo Wang, "Psychological Perspectives on the Changing Nature of Retirement," *American Psychologist* 66 (2011): 170–79.

13. Reuben Ng, Heather G. Allore, Joan K. Monin, and Becca R. Levy, "Retirement as Meaningful: Positive Retirement Stereotypes Associated with Longevity," *Journal of Social Issues* 72, no. 1 (2016): 69–85.

14. Shultz and Wang, "Psychological Perspectives," 170–79.

15. Toni C. Antonucci, Kira S. Birditt, and Hiroko Akiyama, "Convoys of Social Relations: An Interdisciplinary Approach," in *Handbook of Theories of Aging*, ed. Vern L. Bengtson, Merril Silverstein, Norella M. Putney, and Daphna Gans (New York: Springer, 2009), 247–60.

Chapter 12. Making Life Easier for Those Who Someday Will Take Care of You

1. Jolene Brackey, *Creating Moments of Joy for the Person with Alzheimer's or Dementia* (West Lafayette, IN: Purdue University Press, 2007), 158.

2. Ibid., 161.

3. Nancy L. Mace and Peter V. Rabins, *The 36-Hour Day*, 6th ed. (Baltimore: Johns Hopkins University Press, 2017), 7.

4. Barry Stringfellow, "Visiting Physician Sheds New Light on Lyme Disease," *Martha's Vineyard Times*, July 13, 2016, emphasis mine.

5. Alison Bonaguro, "Kris Kristofferson's Wife Talks about Misdiagnosis of Lyme Disease—It Took Integrative Doctor to Connect the Dots," *CMT News*, July 8, 2016.

6. Margery D. Rosen, "8 Treatable Conditions That Mimic Dementia," *AARP Bulletin*, April 2014, www.aarp.org/health/brain-health/info-2014/treatable-conditions-that -mimic-dementia.html.

7. Hai Kang, Fengqing Zhao, Llbo You, Cinzia Giorgetta, Venkatesh D, Sujit Sarkhel, and Ravi Prakash, "Pseudo-dementia: A Neuropsychological Review," *Annals of Indian Academy of Neurology* 17 (2014): 147–54.

8. Centers for Disease Control and Prevention, "Depression Is Not a Normal Part of Growing Older," *Healthy Aging*, updated in 2015, www.cdc.gov/aging/mentalhealth /depression.htm.

9. Walter A. Brown, "Pseudodementia: Issues in Diagnosis," *Psychiatric Times*, April 9, 2005, www.psychiatrictimes.com/dementia/pseudodementia-issues-diagnosis.

10. Robert L. Maher Jr., Joseph T. Hanlon, and Emily R. Hajjar, "Clinical Consequences of Polypharmacy in Elderly," *Expert Opinions on Drug Safety* 13, no. 1 (January 2014): 57.

11. Ibid., 57–65.

12. "Reduced Antipsychotics Recommended for Dementia," *National Psychologist* 25, no. 4 (July/August 2016): 17. "The American Psychiatric Association's released, revised guidelines in May for the limited 'judicious use' of antipsychotic drugs to treat agitation or psychosis in patients with dementia" are summarized in this independent newspaper for practitioners.

13. Atul Gawande, *Being Mortal* (New York: Henry Holt, 2014), 105–6.

14. Ibid., 106.

15. Ibid., 108.

16. Mace and Rabins, *36-Hour Day*, 372.

17. Susan Fletcher, "The Marriage Counselor," *AARP Bulletin* 57, no. 4 (May 2016): 26, emphasis in the original.

18. Mace and Rabins, *36-Hour Day*, 397, 157, 158.

19. Ibid., 157–58.

20. Winnie Hu, "Too Old for Sex? Not at This Nursing Home," *New York Times*, July 12, 2016.

21. Brackey, *Creating Moments of Joy*, 126–27.

22. Ibid., 41.

23. Ibid., 87.

24. Cleveland Clinic Wellness Editors, "Nine Ways to Boost Your Brain Health," *Healthy Memory*, March 28, 2012, www.clevelandclinicwellness.com/body /healthymemory/Pages/9-Ways-to-Boost-Your-Brain-Health.aspx.

25. Henry S. Lodge, *Younger Next Year: The New Science of Aging* (Advise and Consent; PBS Distribution, 2011), DVD.

26. Toni C. Antonucci, James A. Ashton-Miller, Sara Konrath, Joyce M. Lee, Jennifer Brant, Emily B. Falk, et al., "The Right to Move: A Multidisciplinary Lifespan Conceptual Framework," *Current Gerontology and Geriatrics Research*, December 2012, 1–11.

27. Bronnie Ware, *The Top Five Regrets of the Dying* (Australia: Hay House, 2012), vii.

28. Abraham Maslow, *Toward a Psychology of Being* (New York: Wiley, 1968), 206.

29. Samantha J. Heintzelman and Laura A. King, "Life Is Pretty Meaningful," *American Psychologist* 69, no. 6 (September 2014): 569. In this article, the authors give

a more complete quote from Abraham Maslow that I quoted and cited above: "The human needs a framework of values, a philosophy of life . . . in about the same sense that he needs sunlight, calcium, and love."

30. Tyler J. VanderWeele, Shanshan Li, Alexander C. Tsai, and Ichiro Kawachi, "Association between Religious Service Attendance and Lower Suicide Rates among US Women," 73, no. 8 (August 1, 2016): 845–51, analyzes the health data of 89,708 women over a period of 14 years. The researchers report that "compared with women who never participated in religious services, women who attended any religious service once a week or more were five times less likely to commit suicide . . . [And] among devout Catholic women—those in church more than once a week—suicide was essentially nonexistent."

31. Aaron Kheriaty, *The Catholic Guide to Depression* (Bedford, NH: Sophia Press, 2012). Kheriaty is quoted by Melissa Healy in an article in the *LA Times*: "Church Attendance Linked with Reduced Suicide Risk, Especially for Catholics, Study Says," *LA Times*, June 29, 2016.

32. Viktor Frankl, *Man's Search for Meaning* (Boston: Beacon Press, 2014), 150. Published first in Germany in 1946, new editions were published in 1959, 1962, 1984, 1992, and this gift edition by Beacon Press in 2014.

33. Ibid., 153. William J. Winslade, in the afterword, summarizes key teachings and provides updated biographical information on Viktor Frankl.

34. Rosalynn Carter, "Gift of Speech: Remarks of Rosalynn Carter, Honorary Chair of Last Acts" (speech given at Sweet Briar College, February 13, 1997).

Index